WILDERNESS & TRAVEL MEDICINE

ADVENTURE MEDICAL KITS

WILDERNESS & TRAVEL
MEDICINE   A Comprehensive Guide

4th Edition

- *Prepare for adventurous travel*
- *Learn over 50 improvised techniques*
- *Be safe—and confident!*

Eric A. Weiss, M.D., F.A.C.E.P.

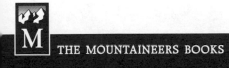

THE MOUNTAINEERS BOOKS

This book is dedicated to Amy and Danny Weiss.
It is also dedicated to my mother and father, for their steadfast
and unselfish support and unconditional love. ↷

 THE MOUNTAINEERS BOOKS
is the nonprofit publishing arm of The Mountaineers,
an organization founded in 1906 and dedicated to the exploration,
preservation, and enjoyment of outdoor and wilderness areas.

1001 SW Klickitat Way, Suite 201, Seattle, WA 98134

© 2012 Adventure Medical Kits
All rights reserved

Fourth edition: first printing 2012, second printing 2013, third printing 2014, fourth
printing 2015, fifth printing 2016

Copy Editor: Heath Lynn Silberfeld / enough said
Cover, Design, and Layout: Peggy Egerdahl
Illustrators: Gray Mouse Graphics, Moore Creative Designs, Rod Nickell, Danny Sun,
    Butch Collier, and Patricia A. Jacobs

Cover photograph: *Climbing El Pico de Orizaba in Mexico*
    © Daniel H. Bailey/Corbis

Library of Congress Cataloging-in-Publication Data
Wilderness & travel medicine : a comprehensive guide / Eric A. Weiss.—4th ed.
p. cm.
Rev. ed. of: Comprehensive guide to wilderness and travel medicine / Eric A. Weiss. 1992.
Includes bibliographical references and index.
ISBN 978-1-59485-658-7 (pbk.)—ISBN 978-1-59485-659-4 (ebook)   1. Outdoor
    medical emergencies—Handbooks, manuals, etc. 2.   Travel—Health aspects—
    Handbooks, manuals, etc. I. Weiss, Eric A., M.D. Comprehensive guide to wilderness
    and travel medicine. II. Title. III. Title: Wilderness and travel medicine.
RC88.9.H55W45 2012
613.6'8—dc23   2011046161

CONTENTS

PREFACE

This book goes far beyond traditional first aid and empowers you to provide "advanced care" when you can't simply call 911. It combines more than twenty-five years of research, clinical experience, and teaching in a powerful guide for those who travel far from modern civilization. Revolutionary advances in emergency medicine knowledge, techniques, and equipment, as well as a new standard of first-aid practice, permeate the text and provide the foundation for laypeople to provide vital emergency care in remote settings.

This book is also unique in that it includes improvised techniques for treating specific injuries and illnesses. It provides creative solutions for fabricating bandages, splints, and even medication from whatever is at hand.

The information in these pages is intended to help you manage medical emergencies in remote environments when professional medical care or rescue is not readily available. It is not a substitute for taking a comprehensive first-aid or wilderness medicine course, or for seeking prompt medical care in the event of an illness or accident. Whenever someone becomes ill or injured, obtaining professional medical attention should take priority after administering appropriate first aid.

The reader should use this book for guidance in difficult and remote situations only and should not attempt to perform any procedure that he or she is not comfortable with or trained to render, unless the victim will die without that intervention. Legally, rescuers are always liable for their own actions and should never take any unnecessary risk or perform any medical procedure unless absolutely necessary.

Consult your physician concerning any medication that you carry, and inquire about potential complications or side effects. Make sure you are not allergic to any drugs that you may use. Sharing your medications with others is potentially dangerous and is not recommended.

Remember, the value of any first-aid book or medical kit is both enhanced and limited by the ability of the owner to use the information and contents effectively and creatively. Taking a Wilderness First Aid (WFA) course, Wilderness First Responder (WFR) course, Emergency Medical Technician (EMT) certification course, or Wilderness and Expedition Medicine Advanced Provider (WEMAP) course—and practicing your skills before you leave home—will better prepare you to manage an emergency when it occurs.

There are also other excellent wilderness medicine educational courses offered that will greatly enhance your knowledge and skill and prepare you for medical care in the backcountry or another austere environment. See www.wilderness-medicine.com

The author and publisher disclaim any liability for injuries, disability, or death that may result from the use of the information in this book, correct or otherwise, or the products in any Adventure Medical Kit.

May all of your journeys be safe, healthy, and filled with adventure!

ACKNOWLEDGMENTS

It is with gratitude and appreciation that I acknowledge and thank my colleagues and friends who have shared my passion for wilderness medicine. Their experience, wisdom, and devotion to wilderness medicine are reflected in many parts of this book. In particular, I extend my gratitude and appreciation for their companionship, inspiration, and guidance to Howard Donner, M.D.; Lanny Johnson, FNP/PA; Peter Hackett, M.D.; Gene Allred, M.D.; Robert Norris, M.D.; Findlay Russell, M.D.; Joe Serra, M.D.; Henry Herrman, D.D.S.; Jim Bagian, M.D.; Tim Erickson, M.D.; Paul Auerbach, M.D.; Robert (Brownie) Schoene, M.D.; Karen Van Hoesen, M.D.; Luanne Freer, M.D.; Richard Clark, M.D.; Ken Zafren, M.D.; Bernard Dannenberg, M.D.; Gary Kibbee; Philip White; Sheryl Olson; and David Breashears.

Eric A. Weiss, M.D., F.A.C.E.P.

WILDERNESS AND TRAVEL MEDICINE

Diagnosis of an injury or illness relies on the ability of the rescuer to examine the victim thoroughly and identify signs and symptoms, which are important medical clues.

Signs and Symptoms

Signs are what you observe when you examine a victim with your eyes, ears, nose, and hands. For example, you might see bluish discoloration of the skin, hear labored or noisy breathing, smell pus in a wound infection, or feel swelling under the skin.

Symptoms are what the victim is experiencing, such as pain, nausea, dizziness, or headache.

In the wilderness, one must utilize whatever supplies or materials are on hand and depend heavily on common sense. Throughout the text you will find features entitled "Weiss Advice," which describe improvised wilderness medicine techniques. Most of these recommendations are supported by research published in medical journals. However, some are merely anecdotal, based on my own personal experience and training.

Another common feature is the "When to Worry" boxes, which help the reader identify situations in which immediate evacuation from the wilderness is recommended. These are only general guidelines, however, and ultimately the circumstance, combined with your own resources, training, and experience, should dictate your actions. When in doubt, it is always better to get out and seek help rather than wait and see what happens.

TRAUMATIC INJURIES AND WHERE TO BEGIN
The Three ABCs

Nine immediate priorities are part of wilderness medicine, regardless of the injury. "Three ABCs" is a helpful mantra for recalling the nine priorities in the order that they are performed. The Three ABCs delineate a rapid evaluation of the scene and the patient in which life-threatening conditions, such as a blocked airway, severe bleeding, or cardiac arrest, are recognized and immediate treatment is rendered.

The Three ABCs of Wilderness First Response
A1　Assess the scene
A2　Airway (Ensure an open airway)
A3　Alert others
B1　Barriers (Protect rescuer with gloves, mask)
B2　Begin CPR if indicated
B3　Bleeding (Stop bleeding)
C1　Complete a secondary survey
C2　Cervical spine protection (Prevent unnecessary movement of the head and neck, protect the spine)
C3　Cover and protect the victim

A1: Assess the Scene

Assess the scene for further hazards to yourself or to the victim—such as rockfall, avalanche, or dangerous animals—before rendering any first-aid care. The worst thing you can do is create another victim or become one yourself. Avoid approaching the victim from directly above if a rock or snowslide is possible. Do not allow your sense of urgency to transform an accident into a risky and foolish rescue attempt.

A2: Airway

Make sure the victim is breathing and does not have an obstructed airway. Speak loudly to the victim as you approach. A response indicates that the victim is breathing and has a pulse. For infants and children, call their name and gently tap their hands and feet. If the victim is unresponsive, immediately determine if he is breathing. If he is facedown, logroll him onto his back so that the head, shoulders, and torso move as a single unit without twisting (**Figs. 1 & 2**).

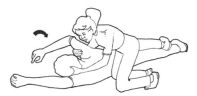

Fig. 1　*Single rescuer logrolling a victim faceup without twisting the spine*

Logrolling a victim with Multiple Rescuers

If the victim must be rolled or turned to place insulation or a spine board under him, or if he is vomiting, logroll him with the head and body held as a unit (**Fig. 2a–d**). In the event of a suspected spine injury, it is generally better to send for professional rescue assistance than to attempt to transport the victim yourself.

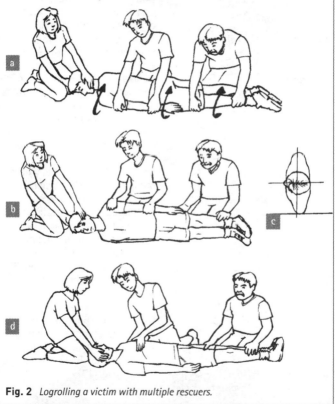

Fig. 2 *Logrolling a victim with multiple rescuers.*

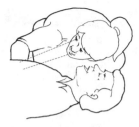

Fig. 3 *Checking for breathing*

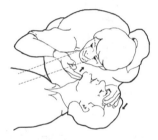

Fig. 4 *Opening the airway of an unconscious victim when trauma is not suspected*

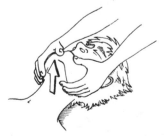

Fig. 5 *Using the jaw-thrust technique to open the airway after trauma*

Place your ear and cheek close to the victim's mouth and nose to detect air movement, while looking for movement of the chest and abdomen (**Fig. 3**). In cold weather, look for a vapor cloud and feel for warm air movement.

If the victim is not breathing, or has noisy (obstructed) breathing, open the airway (**Fig. 4**). The most common reason for an airway obstruction in an unconscious trauma victim is relaxation of the muscles of the tongue and throat, which allows the tongue to fall back and block the airway. Use the jaw-thrust technique to open the airway when trauma is suspected. It minimizes movement of the neck, which is potentially hazardous if the victim has a spine injury. The jaw thrust is performed by getting on your knees behind the victim's head, placing your hands on either side of the victim's jawbone, and pulling the base of the jaw up and forward (**Fig. 5**). If you do not detect breathing after opening the airway or observe only occasional gasps (agonal respiration), presume that the victim is in cardiac arrest, immediately alert others, and quickly initiate CPR (see "B2: Begin CPR if Indicated," page 19).

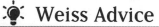 Weiss Advice

Opening the Airway with Two Safety Pins

Keeping the airway open with the jaw-thrust technique ties up your hands. If you are by yourself, an airway can be kept open by pinning the front of the victim's tongue to the lower lip with two safety pins (**Fig. 6a**).

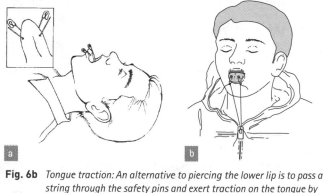

Fig. 6b *Tongue traction: An alternative to piercing the lower lip is to pass a string through the safety pins and exert traction on the tongue by securing the end of the string to the victim's shirt button or jacket zipper.*

A3: Alert Others
Before becoming more involved with the resuscitation, take a few seconds to call or send someone for help and to alert others to the accident.

B1: Barriers
Any time blood or bodily fluids are present, it is important to protect yourself from blood-, urine-, and saliva-borne germs, such as hepatitis and HIV. The CDC estimates that more than one million people are living with HIV in the United States. One in five (21 percent) of those people

living with HIV is unaware of their infection. And the risk of infectious hepatitis is far greater. Protect your hands with virus-proof gloves and use a barrier device when performing mouth-to-mouth rescue breathing. Even nitrile gloves can leak, so make sure you wash your hands or wipe them with an antimicrobial towelette after removing the gloves.

WARNING: Many people are allergic to latex. Latex allergies can produce skin rashes, severe anaphylactic reactions, and death. If you suspect that you might have an allergy to latex, use powder-free nitrile gloves.

Weiss Advice

Improvised Barrier

Using any gloves is better than using your bare hands. Dishwashing gloves make an effective barrier to blood. An improvised glove can also be made by placing your hand inside a sandwich or garbage bag and securing it to your wrist with tape or string.

Weiss Advice

Improvised Barrier for Mouth-to-Mouth Breathing

A glove can be modified and used as a barrier shield when performing rescue breathing (**Fig. 7a-c**). Simply cut the middle finger of the glove at its halfway point and insert the glove into the victim's mouth. Stretch the glove across the victim's mouth and blow into it as you would to inflate a balloon. The slit creates a one-way valve, preventing backflow of the victim's saliva.

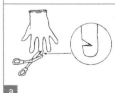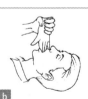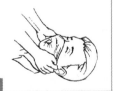

Fig. 7 Improvised glove barrier

B2: Begin CPR if Indicated

Recognition of cardiac arrest is not always a simple matter for untrained rescuers. If a victim is unresponsive with no breathing or no normal breathing (i.e., only gasping) after opening the airway, immediately begin CPR. Early CPR can improve the likelihood of survival, especially if followed by rapid defibrillation with an automated external defibrillator (AED).

Trained rescuers should take no more than 10 seconds (30 seconds if the victim is severely hypothermic) to check for a pulse. Place your index and middle fingers on the victim's throat over the Adam's apple, then slide your fingers down the side of the victim's neck to the space between the Adam's apple and neck muscle to feel the carotid pulse (**Fig. 8**). If you do not detect a pulse, initiate CPR (see "Life-Threatening Emergencies: Cardiopulmonary Resuscitation," page 22).

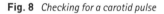

Fig. 8 *Checking for a carotid pulse*

If the patient does not breathe spontaneously after establishing an airway, then begin mouth-to-mouth rescue breathing (see "Rescue Breathing," page 25).

B3: Bleeding

Check the victim for signs of profuse bleeding. With a gloved or protected hand, feel inside any clothing and check underneath the victim for signs of bleeding. To stop bleeding, use your gloved hand to apply pressure directly to the wound (**Fig. 9**). If bleeding from

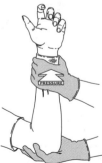

Fig. 9 *To stop bleeding, use your gloved hand to apply pressure directly to the wound.*

How to Apply a Tourniquet

1. Tourniquet material should be wide and flat, to prevent crushing tissue. Use a firm bandage, belt, or strap that is 8–10 cm (3 to 4 inches) wide and will not stretch. Never use wire, rope, or any material that will cut the skin.
2. Wrap the bandage snugly around the extremity several times as close above the wound as possible, and tie an overhand knot.
3. Place a stick or similar object on the knot and tie another overhand knot over the stick.
4. Twist the stick until the bandage becomes tight enough to stop the bleeding. Tie or tape the stick in place to prevent it from unraveling.
5. Mark the victim with the letters "TK," and note the time the tourniquet was applied.
6. If you are more than an hour from medical care, at the end of one hour, while maintaining direct pressure on the wound, loosen the tourniquet very slowly. If bleeding is still heavy, retighten the tourniquet. If bleeding is manageable with direct pressure alone, leave the tourniquet in place, but do not tighten it again unless severe bleeding starts.

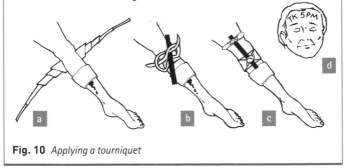

Fig. 10 *Applying a tourniquet*

an extremity cannot be stopped by direct pressure and the victim is in danger of bleeding to death, apply a tourniquet. (**Fig.10a–d**) (A tourniquet is any band applied around an arm or leg so tightly that all blood flow beyond the band is cut off.) If the tourniquet is left on for more than 4 hours, the arm or leg beyond the tourniquet may die and require amputation. Damage to the arm or leg is rare if the tourniquet is left on less than 2 hours.

In the face of massive extremity hemorrhage, it is better to accept the risk of damage to the limb than to have a victim bleed to death (see "Wounds: Cuts and Abrasions," page 102).

The Combat-Application-Tourniquet (C-A-T), www.combattourniquet .com is a small and lightweight one-handed tourniquet that is used by the U.S. military. Combined with a one-handed windlass system, the C-A-T uses a self-adhering band and a friction adaptor buckle to fit a wide range of extremities. The windlass uses a free-moving internal band to provide true circumferential pressure to an extremity. The windlass is then locked in place; this requires only one hand, with a Windlass Clip.

C1: Complete a Secondary Survey

Once you have ensured that no life-threatening issues are present, perform a head-to-toe examination of the victim, looking for further evidence of injury. Gently push on every part of the victim, assessing for pain, swelling, or deformity.

C2: Cervical Spine Protection

The spinal cord is vital for life. It runs through the cervical vertebrae in the neck. Spinal cord damage can cause permanent paralysis or death. It is necessary to immobilize the head, neck, and torso after an accident that could have broken the victim's neck, such as a fall, head injury, or diving injury, and if any of the following are present:

- The victim is unconscious.
- The victim complains of neck or back pain.
- There is tenderness in the back of the neck or upper back when touched.
- There is numbness, tingling, or altered sensation in the extremities.
- The victim is unable to move or has weakness in an arm or leg not due to direct trauma to that part.
- The victim has an altered level of consciousness or is under the influence of drugs or alcohol.
- The victim has another very painful injury that may distract him from the pain in his neck, such as a thigh (femur) or pelvis fracture, dislocated shoulder, or broken rib.

If a cervical spine injury is suspected, the rescuer should immobilize the victim's head and neck and prevent any movement of the torso (see "Treatment of Specific Fractures: Neck and Spine," page 75). Do not move the victim with a suspected spine injury from a safe location. The victim should be evacuated by professional rescuers.

C3: Cover and Protect the Victim

If it is cold, place insulating garments or blankets underneath and on top of the victim for protection from hypothermia. Remove and replace any wet clothing. If it is hot, loosen the victim's clothing and create shade. If the victim is in a dangerous area, move him to a safer location while, if indicated, maintaining spine immobilization.

ORGANIZING A RESCUE TEAM

In the wilderness, developing a team approach at the site of the accident is vital to the success of the rescue. Begin by designating a leader. This individual can be the climb leader, head boatman, or anyone who assumes the leadership role. When possible, this person should direct all first-aid efforts and delegate duties, rather than perform them. If the leader becomes intimately involved in a specific function, he loses the ability to maintain a team effort. The leader should evaluate the victim's injuries, party size, and terrain and then develop a plan for either evacuating the patient or obtaining professional assistance.

LIFE-THREATENING EMERGENCIES: CPR, RESCUE BREATHING, CHOKING/OBSTRUCTED AIRWAY

Cardiopulmonary Resuscitation (CPR)

New guidelines by the American Heart Association recommend that the three steps of cardiopulmonary resuscitation (CPR) be rearranged. The new first step is doing chest compressions instead of mouth-to-mouth breathing. The new guidelines apply to adults, children, and infants but exclude newborns.

When to Start and Stop CPR

Do not be afraid to start CPR, fearing that you might be criticized for not continuing it indefinitely. An old saying in medicine is "Once started, CPR should never be stopped in the field." Adhering to this dictum is not only impractical but also potentially hazardous to the rescuers. It is well established—when an AED for defibrillation is not readily available—that if victims do not respond after 10 to 15 minutes of CPR, they never will. The only rare exceptions have been victims who were severely hypothermic. It may be better to give the victim the benefit of the doubt and start CPR, even if no heartbeat or breath has been detected for a prolonged time. It is difficult to know exactly how long a person found unconscious has actually been in cardiac arrest.

CPR: Adult and Child (Older than One Year)

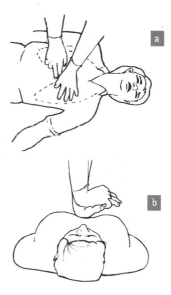

1. If you find an unresponsive victim (i.e., no movement or response to stimulation) or witness an individual who suddenly collapses, attempt to wake him by tapping on his shoulder and shouting at him. If breathing is absent or only occasionally gasping, assume the victim is in cardiac arrest. If you are trained in how to detect a pulse, take no more than 10 seconds to check for one (30 seconds if the victim is severely hypothermic) and, if you do not definitely feel a pulse within that time, start chest compressions.

2. Place the victim on his back on a firm surface. Place the heel of your hand in the middle of his chest. Put your other hand on top of the first with your fingers interlaced (**Fig. 11a & b**).

Fig. 11

Place the heel of one hand in the middle of the chest. Place the other hand on top with fingers interlaced. Your shoulders should line up directly over the victim's breastbone.

3. Compress the chest at least 5 cm (2 inches). Allow the chest to completely recoil before the next compression. (Your shoulders should line up directly over the victim's breastbone, with elbows straight.)

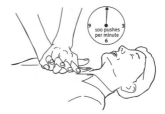

4. Keeping your arms stiff and using a smooth motion, compress the breastbone at a rate of at least 100 pushes per minute. (That's about the same rhythm as the beat of the Bee Gees' song "Stayin' Alive.") (**Fig. 12**). Do not remove your hands from the victim's chest between compressions. You may feel pops and snaps when you first begin chest compressions— don't stop! You're not going to make the victim worse.

Fig. 12 *Keep arms stiff and compress the breastbone at a rate of at least 100 pushes per minute.*

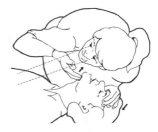

5. After 30 compressions, open the victim's airway using the head-tilt, chin-lift method (**Fig. 13**).

Fig. 13 *Opening the airway*

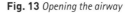

Pinch the victim's nose, and make a seal over the victim's mouth with yours. Use a CPR mask if available, or improvise one from materials at hand (see Weiss Advice, page 18). Give the victim a breath big enough to make the chest rise. Let the chest fall, then repeat the rescue breath once more. If the chest doesn't rise on the first breath, reposition the head and try again. If you don't feel comfortable with this step, continue to do chest compressions at a rate of at least 100 per minute without rescue breathing (hands-only CPR).

6. Use a compression-to-breathing ratio of 30 chest compressions for every two breaths.
7. If two rescuers are working together, switch off doing compressions and breathing every 2 minutes to prevent fatigue. Check every 5 minutes for the return of a pulse or spontaneous breathing.
8. If you have access to an AED, continue to do CPR until you can attach it to the victim and turn it on. After turning on the AED, follow the prompts. If a shock is administered, reassess the victim for return of a pulse and breathing. If there is no change, resume chest compressions immediately after the shock.

CPR: Infant (Younger than One Year)

1. Try to wake the infant by rubbing the soles or tapping on the shoulder or chest. Do not shake a baby.
2. If the baby is not breathing, put two fingers on the breastbone directly between the baby's nipples. Push straight down about 4 cm (1.5 inches) or about one-third of the thickness of the baby's chest, then let the chest rise all the way back up. Do this 30 times, about twice per second.
3. After pushing on the chest 30 times, cover the baby's entire mouth and nose with your mouth and gently blow until you see the chest rise. Let the air escape—the chest will go back down—and give one more breath.
4. Continue the compression-to-breathing ratio of 30 compressions for every two breaths.
5. Don't stop until the baby wakes up or starts breathing independently.

Rescue Breathing

Rescue Breathing: Adult

1. Check for breathing (see "A2: Airway," page 14). If the victim is not lying faceup, gently logroll the entire body over while maintaining spine precautions (see **Figs. 1 & 2**, pages 14 & 15).
2. If no breathing is detected, open the airway with the head-tilt maneuver. Place the palm of one hand on the forehead, then tilt

the head back while the fingers of the other hand grasp and lift the chin (**Fig. 13**).

Note: If a neck injury is suspected, use the jaw-thrust technique to open the airway (**Fig. 5,** page 16). Sweep two fingers through the victim's mouth to remove any foreign material or broken teeth.

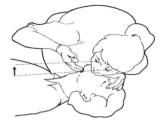

Fig. 14 *Rescue breathing, adult*

3. If the victim does not start to breathe spontaneously, pinch the nostrils closed and place your mouth over the victim's mouth (**Fig. 14**). A CPR Microshield barrier or modified glove (see Weiss Advice, page 18) can be used during mouth-to-mouth rescue breathing to prevent physical contact with the victim's mouth.

4. Blow air into the victim until you see the chest rise. Remove your mouth to allow the victim to exhale. Give two breaths.

5. Repeat this procedure, giving a vigorous breath every 5 seconds until the victim starts to breathe spontaneously, help arrives, or you are too exhausted to continue.

6. If air does not move in and out of the victim's mouth easily or if the chest does not rise, try tilting the head farther back or, if a cervical spine injury is suspected, repeat the jaw-thrust technique, pushing the victim's jaw farther out. If breathing still does not occur, the airway may be obstructed by a foreign body (see "Choking/Obstructed Airway," page 28).

7. During mouth-to-mouth rescue breathing, the victim's stomach will often fill with air, eventually resulting in vomiting. If vomiting occurs, logroll the victim in a manner that maintains spine alignment (**Fig. 15a & b**), then clear the airway.

Rescue Breathing: Child (Older than One Year)

1. Cover the child's mouth with your mouth. Pinch the child's nose closed with the thumb and forefinger of your hand that is on the

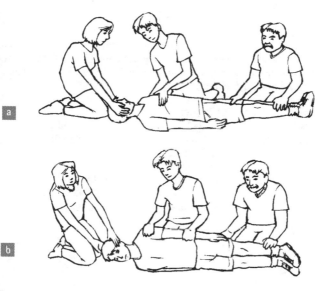

Fig. 15 *Logrolling a victim onto their side for vomiting or to place a board or insulation under the victim.*

forehead for the head tilt. Use your other hand to lift the chin (**Fig. 16**).

2. Breathe two slow breaths (1 to 1.5 seconds) into the child's mouth, with a 2-second pause between breaths. Breathe in enough air to make the child's chest rise.

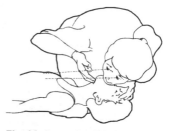

Fig. 16 *Rescue breathing, child*

Choking/Obstructed Airway

Choking is a life-threatening emergency that occurs when something blocks the victim's airway so that he cannot breathe. Choking most often occurs when someone is eating. Choking should be suspected when an individual suddenly becomes agitated and clutches the throat, especially while eating. The victim may be unable to speak and then may become cyanotic (turn blue).

Choking: Adult and Child (Heimlich Maneuver)

1. Stand behind the victim and wrap your arms around the victim's waist. Make a fist with one of your hands, then place it just above the victim's navel and below the rib cage, with the thumb side against the victim's abdomen.
2. Grasp your fist with your other hand and pull it forcefully toward you, into the victim's abdomen and slightly upward, with a quick thrust. If unsuccessful, repeat the procedure (**Fig. 17**).

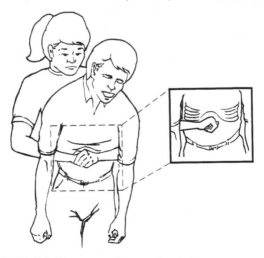

Fig. 17 *Heimlich maneuver for a standing victim*

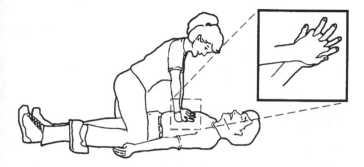

Fig. 18 *Heimlich maneuver for an unconscious adult*

If the adult or child becomes unconscious:

1. Lay the victim faceup and attempt rescue breathing (see "Rescue Breathing," page 25).
2. If you cannot get air into the victim and/or the chest does not rise with rescue breathing, perform the Heimlich maneuver while kneeling and straddling the victim's thighs. Use the heel of your hand instead of your fist (**Fig. 18**).
3. If still unsuccessful, look for foreign material in the victim's mouth and, if found, remove it. Continue to perform the Heimlich maneuver and periodically attempt rescue breathing. If multiple attempts at clearing the airway and breathing air into the patient are unsuccessful, a cricothyroidotomy (surgical airway) is indicated.

Cricothyroidotomy (Surgical Airway)

A cricothyroidotomy is a technique that allows rapid entrance into the air passage in a victim who is unable to breathe from a blocked airway. It is a very challenging and potentially complication-prone procedure, but it may be lifesaving. It should be attempted only after the Heimlich maneuver and other noninvasive techniques to relieve the obstruction in the airway have been exhausted, and the victim is on the verge of dying from lack of air.

In the wilderness, a cricothyroidotomy is done by cutting a hole in the thin cricothyroid membrane of the windpipe (trachea) and then placing a hollow object into the trachea to let air enter the lungs. The cricothyroid membrane lies just below the Adam's apple in the center of the neck and feels like a small depression between the Adam's apple and the firm ring below it (the cricoid cartilage).

How to Perform a Cricothyroidotomy

1. With the victim lying faceup, clean the neck around the Adam's apple with an antiseptic if one is readily available. Put on protective gloves.

2. Find the Adam's apple with your finger (this is the most prominent firm structure in the center of the neck). Slowly run your finger downward toward the chest (keep your finger in the midline of the neck as you do this) until you feel a small indentation between the bottom of the Adam's apple and the top of the cricoid cartilage (the next firm and prominent structure that you feel as you move down the neck). The indentation between the Adam's apple and the cricoid cartilage in the windpipe is called

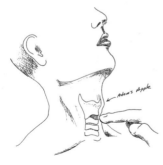

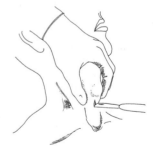

Fig. 19 *Location of the cricothyroid membrane just below the Adam's apple in the midline of the neck.*

Fig. 20 *Making a vertical 2.5 cm (1-inch) incision through the skin over the cricothyroid membrane.*

the cricothyroid membrane and is the spot that you want to puncture (**Fig. 19**).

3. Make a vertical 2.5 cm (1-inch) incision with a knife through the skin over the membrane (go a little bit above and below the membrane) while using the fingers of your other hand to pry the skin edges apart. Anticipate bleeding from the wound. After the skin is cut apart, puncture the membrane by stabbing it with your knife or other pointy object (**Fig. 20**).

4. While stabilizing the windpipe between the fingers of one hand, with your other hand insert (through the membrane) a hollow object—such as the barrel of a syringe (see below), the casing of a ballpoint pen, or a stiff straw (**Fig. 20–22**). Secure the object in place with tape.

5. Breathe air into the victim through the object, as if you were blowing through a straw, and then remove your mouth to allow exhaled air to exit. Repeat this step at the same frequency as if you were performing mouth-to-mouth rescue breathing.

☀ Weiss Advice

Using a Syringe as a Breathing Tube

Remove the plunger from the barrel of a 1-cc or 3-cc syringe. Using a sharp knife or saw, cut the barrel at a 45-degree angle at its midpoint to create an improvised airway for inserting through the cricothyroid membrane (**Fig. 21 & 22**).

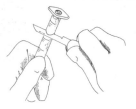

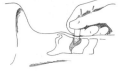

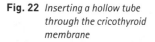

Fig. 21 *Cutting the barrel of a 1-cc or 3-cc syringe at a 45° angle*

Fig. 22 *Inserting a hollow tube through the cricothyroid membrane*

SHOCK

Shock is a life-threatening condition in which blood flow to the tissues of the body is inadequate and cells are deprived of oxygen. Any serious injury or illness can produce shock. Examples are severe internal or external bleeding (hemorrhagic shock), bleeding due to a thigh (femur) or pelvis fracture, major burns, dehydration, heart failure (cardiogenic shock), severe allergic reactions (anaphylactic shock), severe infections (septic shock), and spinal cord injuries with paralysis (neurogenic shock).

Signs and Symptoms

The skin may be pale, cool, or clammy. The pulse is weak and rapid or even undetectable. (In shock produced by a spinal cord injury, the pulse will remain normal or slow.) Breathing may be shallow, rapid, or irregular. Mental status may be altered (the victim may be confused, restless, or combative).

Treatment

It is important to recognize shock and to transport the victim to a medical facility immediately.

1. Keep the victim lying down, covered, warm, and insulated from the ground.
2. Stop any obvious signs of bleeding.
3. Loosen any restrictive clothing.
4. Splint all broken bones. If the femur bone is fractured, apply and maintain traction (see Weiss Advice, page 87). If a pelvic fracture is suspected, apply a pelvic wrap (see **Figs. 38 & 39**, page 85).
5. Elevate the legs so that gravity can help improve the blood supply to the heart and brain only if the victim has fainted or is in shock from external bleeding that has been controlled. For internal bleeding, avoid unnecessary movement and keep the victim lying flat. For heart failure shock, the victim may be more comfortable with head and shoulders raised slightly.

HEAD INJURIES

Head trauma and traumatic brain injury (TBI) are caused by a bump, blow, or jolt to the head or body that causes the head and brain to move back and forth quickly. When the head hits a hard object such as a boulder, the impact can fracture the skull, bruise the brain, or cause severe bleeding inside the brain from damaged blood vessels. Shearing forces from sudden deceleration of the brain against the inside of the skull can also tear blood vessels on the surface of the brain, leading to an expanding blood clot and pressure on the brain (intracranial pressure).

Rising intracranial pressure is bad for several reasons. The increased pressure makes it difficult for the heart to pump enough blood to the head. This is a major catastrophe for the brain, which depends on a constant supply of blood to bring it oxygen and other nutrients. If the pressure within the skull rises high enough, it can force parts of the brain downward through the base of the skull (herniation), causing damage to the brain structures and, ultimately, death. Compression of one of the nerves as the brain swells produces dilatation of one or both pupils, which is an important sign of a severe head injury.

Concussions

(See also "Moderate Head Injury," page 35.)

Concussions are sometimes referred to as mild brain injuries because they are usually not life-threatening. Even so, their effects can be serious, and sport-related concussion is a controversial topic in medicine. A concussion typically results in the rapid onset of short-lived impairment of neurologic function, such as a brief loss of consciousness and/or amnesia for the event. Most victims with a concussion recover quickly and fully. During recovery, many people have a range of symptoms that may appear right away or may not be noticed for hours or even days after the injury (**Table 1**). Wearing a protective helmet can reduce the severity of traumatic brain injury.

Table 1

Possible Symptoms Following a Concussion

Thinking/ Remembering	Physical	Emotional/ Mood	Sleep
Difficulty thinking clearly	Fuzzy or blurry vision	Irritability	Sleeping more than usual
Feeling slowed down	Nausea or vomiting (early on)	Sadness	Sleeping less than usual
Difficulty concentrating	Sensitivity to noise or light	More emotional	Trouble falling asleep
Difficulty remembering new information	Feeling tired, having no energy	Nervousness or anxiety	

Head injuries can be subdivided into different categories based on their severity:

- Severe head injury
- Moderate head injury
- Head injury with no loss of consciousness

Severe Head Injury

Loss of consciousness for more than 5 to 10 minutes or an altered level of consciousness (victim is confused or does not act normally) following a head injury is a sign of significant brain injury. Assess the victim's airway and perform rescue breathing if necessary. Because there is a potential for accompanying neck and spine injuries with severe head trauma, immobilize the victim's spine. Immediately evacuate the victim to a medical facility. During transportation, maintain spine immobilization and keep the victim's head pointed uphill on sloping terrain. Be prepared to logroll the victim onto his side if he vomits. Continually monitor the victim's airway for signs of obstruction (listen for noisy or labored breathing) and a decreasing respiratory rate.

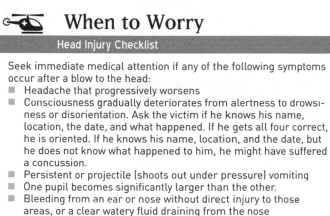

When to Worry

Head Injury Checklist

Seek immediate medical attention if any of the following symptoms occur after a blow to the head:

- Headache that progressively worsens
- Consciousness gradually deteriorates from alertness to drowsiness or disorientation. Ask the victim if he knows his name, location, the date, and what happened. If he gets all four correct, he is oriented. If he knows his name, location, and the date, but he does not know what happened to him, he might have suffered a concussion.
- Persistent or projectile (shoots out under pressure) vomiting
- One pupil becomes significantly larger than the other.
- Bleeding from an ear or nose without direct injury to those areas, or a clear watery fluid draining from the nose
- Bruising behind the ears or around the eyes when there is no direct injury to those areas
- Seizure

Moderate Head Injury

Short-term unconsciousness, in which the victim wakes after a minute or two and gradually regains normal mental status and physical abilities, is evidence of a concussion (see "Concussions," page 33). Amnesia about the event and repetitive questioning by the victim are not uncommon.

To be safe, evacuate the victim to a medical facility for evaluation. At a minimum in the backcountry, keep the victim under close observation for at least 24 hours, and do not allow the victim to perform potentially hazardous activities. Wake the victim from sleep every 3 to 4 hours to check briefly that the condition has not deteriorated and that the victim can be easily aroused. If the victim becomes increasingly lethargic, confused, or combative; is not acting normally; or develops any other signs of concern (see When to Worry, above), evacuate him to a medical center immediately.

Getting plenty of rest and sleep helps the brain to heal. Avoid situations that could produce a subsequent head injury, and consult with a physician before returning to contact sports. A repeat concussion that occurs before the brain has fully healed can be very dangerous and may slow recovery or increase the chance for long-term problems.

Mild Head Injury with No Loss of Consciousness

If an individual hits his head but never loses consciousness, he may still have suffered a mild concussion, but it is usually not serious or life-threatening. He may have a mild headache, bleed from a scalp wound, or have a large bump on his head, but evacuation isn't necessary unless the victim develops any of the problems listed among those on the "Head Injury Checklist."

Skull Fractures

Fracture of the skull is not life-threatening unless associated with underlying brain injury or severe bleeding.

Signs and Symptoms

Signs of a skull fracture include a sensation that the skull is uneven when touching the scalp; blood or clear fluid draining from the ears or nose without direct trauma to those areas; and black-and-blue discoloration around the eyes (raccoon eyes) or behind the ears (Battle's sign).

Treatment

Evacuate the victim to a medical facility as soon as possible.

Scalp Wounds

Scalp lacerations are common after head injuries. They tend to bleed a lot because of their rich blood supply. Fortunately, bleeding can usually be stopped by applying direct pressure to the wound with your gloved hand. It might be necessary to hold pressure for up to 30 minutes.

🔆 Weiss Advice

Hair-Tying a Scalp Wound Closed

If you're faced with a bleeding scalp wound and the injured person has a healthy head of hair, you can tie the wound closed using the victim's own hair (**Fig. 23a & b**). Take a piece of dental floss or sewing thread and lay it on top of, and parallel to, the wound. Twirl a few strands of hair on each side of the wound, then cross them over the wound in opposite directions, forcing the wound edges closed. Have an assistant tie together the strands of hair and the dental floss or thread while you hold the wound closed with the strands of hair. A square knot works best. You can also use a drop of superglue to hold together the strands of hair. Repeat this technique as many times as necessary along the length of the wound until the cut is closed.

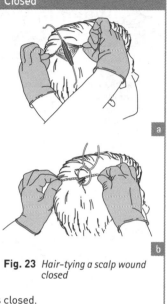

Fig. 23 *Hair-tying a scalp wound closed*

HEADACHE

At least 60 percent of people will have a significant headache at some time in their lives, and it is one of the most common reasons for visiting a physician. Headaches can stem from innumerable causes, including tension and stress, migraine, dehydration, altitude illness (see "Altitude Illness," page 153), alcohol hangover, carbon monoxide poisoning, brain tumor, stroke, aneurysm, intracranial bleed, fever, flu, meningitis and other infectious diseases, high blood pressure, sinus infections, and dental problems. Suddenly going without caffeine during a backpacking trip, especially if you regularly drink more than three cups of coffee a day, can also precipitate a headache.

When to Worry

Headaches

Some headaches may signal a life-threatening illness. Get to a medical facility as soon as possible if you experience any of the following:

- The headache is the worst of your life and came on suddenly and severely (aneurysm or intracranial bleeding).
- Your arms and legs on one side are weak, numb, or paralyzed, or one side of your face appears droopy (stroke).
- You are unable to talk or express yourself clearly (stroke).
- You have a fever, stiff neck, or rash (meningitis).
- Your headache grows steadily worse over time (brain tumor).
- You have repetitive vomiting.
- Seizures or convulsions develop.
- The pain does not go away over a period of 24 hours.

Tension Headache

Tension headache, also known as stress or muscle contraction headache, is the most common type of headache and affects people of all ages. Pain is related to continuous contractions of the muscles of the head and neck and can last from 30 minutes to 7 days.

Signs and Symptoms

The headache is often described as tight or viselike, and it is felt on both sides, especially in the back of the head and neck. The pain is not made worse by walking, climbing, or performing physical activity.

Sensitivity to light may occur, but nausea and vomiting are not usually present.

Treatment

Loosen any tight-fitting pack straps or hat, and adjust your pack so that it rides comfortably. Ibuprofen (Motrin) 600 mg or acetaminophen (Tylenol) 1000 mg may help relieve the discomfort. A neck and scalp massage may be beneficial.

Migraine Headache

The term migraine is often used as a catchall but should be reserved for those headaches that show specific patterns. Migraines are recurrent headaches that usually start during adolescence.

Signs and Symptoms

Migraines typically involve only one side of the head (though they can be experienced on both sides) and are associated with nausea, vomiting, and sensitivity to light. About 15 percent of people with migraine headaches will experience an aura (flashing lights, distorted shapes and colors, blurred vision, or other visual apparitions) prior to the onset of the headache. Walking or physical exertion makes the pain worse.

Treatment

Ibuprofen (Motrin) 800 mg along with caffeinated beverages, such as coffee, may help relieve symptoms, especially if taken early. Stronger prescription medications such as Tylenol with codeine, acetaminophen with hydrocodone (Vicodin), sumatriptan (Imitrex), or eletriptan (Relpax) may be needed. Ondansetron (Zofran) 4 mg oral dissolving tablet will help treat the nausea and vomiting associated with migraine headaches. Lying down in the shade with a cool compress on the forehead may be helpful.

Dehydration Headache

Headache can be an early sign of dehydration.

Signs and Symptoms

The pain of a dehydration headache is felt on both sides of the head and is usually made worse when the victim stands from a lying position.

Treatment

Resting and drinking at least 1–2 L (1–2 quarts) of water should relieve the pain. (On average, one should drink about 4 L (1 gallon) a day when backpacking.) A good barometer of your hydration status is the color of your urine. If it is not clear, like gin, then you're not drinking enough.

Sinus Headache
Signs and Symptoms
Sinus headache is usually associated with a sinus infection and typified by fever, nasal congestion, production of nasal discharge, and pain in the front of the face. Tapping over the sinuses may increase the pain (see "Sinus Infection [Sinusitis]," page 119).

Treatment
Use an oral decongestant (pseudoephedrine [Sudafed]), a nasal spray (phenylephrine [Neo-Synephrine] or oxymetazoline [Afrin]), and an antibiotic (amoxicillin [Augmentin], azithromycin [Zithromax], or erythromycin).

Meningitis
Meningitis is a severe infection that involves the lining of the brain and spinal cord.

Signs and Symptoms
The headache of meningitis is severe and often accompanied by nausea, vomiting, fever, altered level of consciousness (e.g., confusion or bizarre behavior), and a stiff neck. The victim may demonstrate discomfort when the chin is flexed downward against the chest and may complain that the pain also occurs in the back. An infant can suffer meningitis without a stiff neck and may manifest only poor feeding, fever, lethargy, and irritability.

Treatment
If meningitis is suspected, the victim should be started on broad-spectrum antibiotics and evacuated immediately.

EYE
Eye Trauma
Signs and Symptoms
If the eye is hit, a visible layer of blood may settle behind the cornea (clear covering over the front of the eye) during the next 6 to 8 hours.

If the eyeball is perforated, the victim will experience a loss of vision ranging from blurred sight to total blindness. Other signs and symptoms include pain, a dilated and unreactive pupil, and blood in the eye.

Trauma to the eye can also cause the retina to become detached from the back of the eye. Symptoms include persistent flashes of light and floating spots in the field of vision. Vision loss is painless.

Treatment

If the eye is hit, the eye should be patched closed with a gauze pad and tape. Transport the victim immediately to medical care, keeping the head elevated and in an upright position.

If the eye is perforated (ruptured), do not rinse the eye or try to remove any object stuck into the eyeball. Cover the eye with a paper cone, cup, or other protective object and secure this protective covering in place with a bandage so that it does not put pressure on the eye (**Fig. 24a & b**). If possible, patch both eyes or have the victim keep both eyes closed. Evacuate the victim to a medical facility immediately. If evacuation will be delayed more than 6 hours, start antibiotic therapy with penicillin, cephalexin (Keflex), or erythromycin.

A detached retina requires surgical repair. Seek immediate medical care.

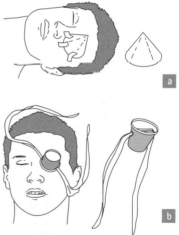

Fig. 24 *Two different techniques for improvising and securing a protective cover for a perforated or ruptured eye.*

Scratched Eye (Corneal Abrasion)

The cornea, the clear covering over the front of the eye, is easily scratched or abraded.

Signs and Symptoms

- The victim will feel as if sand is in the eye.
- The eye will usually appear bloodshot, and tearing and slight blurring of vision are often present.
- Intense pain, made worse by blinking the eyes, may occur.
- The victim is sensitive to light.
- Close inspection of the cornea may show a slight irregularity on its surface.

Treatment

1. Check the eyes carefully for foreign material, making sure to examine under the upper lid.
2. Apply cool compresses to relieve some of the irritation.
3. If available, apply antibiotic drops such as tobramycin (Tobrex) ophthalmic drops for 2 days every 2 to 3 hours while awake.
4. Administer pain medication to the victim.
5. Have the victim rest both eyes as much as possible. Most of the time, the injury heals by itself in a day or two.
6. To reduce pain, patch the eye with an eye patch or a bandage for 24 hours. If an eye patch or other bandage is not available, the eye can be taped closed or the victim can wear sunglasses. Do not patch an eye closed if any sign of infection is present.

When to Worry

Scratched Eye

Seek medical care immediately if the victim has a scratched eye or snow blindness and any of the following signs or symptoms:

- The injury does not heal spontaneously in 2 days.
- Redness, pain, or swelling increases.
- Greenish fluid begins to drain from the eye.
- The victim's vision worsens.

Snow Blindness

Snow blindness is a sunburn to the eye that results in a corneal abrasion. It results from exposure to intense ultraviolet radiation at high altitude or while traveling in the snow. At higher elevations, more ultraviolet light is easily reflected off snow. Because signs and symptoms of snow blindness are delayed by about 4 to 6 hours from the time of exposure to the light, victims are unaware that the injury is occurring until it is too late to prevent it. Wearing adequate eye protection (100 percent UV-blocking sunglasses with side protectors) can prevent snow blindness.

:☀: Weiss Advice

Improvising Sunglasses

It is possible to improvise a pair of "sunglasses" that will help protect eyes from ultraviolet light, especially in snow and at elevations above 2500 m (8000 feet).

Cut small slits in a piece of cardboard (e.g., use one side of a cracker or cereal box) or in a piece of duct tape folded back over onto itself (**Fig. 25**). The slits should be just wide enough to see through, and no larger than the diameter of the eye. Tape or tie these "sunglasses" around the head to minimize the amount of light hitting the eyes.

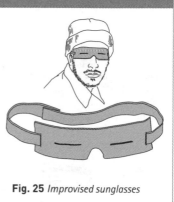

Fig. 25 *Improvised sunglasses*

Signs, Symptoms, and Treatment

The signs, symptoms, and treatment for snow blindness are the same as for a scratched eye (see previous page).

Subconjunctival Hemorrhage

Small blood clots on the white part of the eye sometimes occur after physical exertion, coughing, or strangulation. This is not a serious condition. The hemorrhage will resolve on its own over a few weeks.

Superficial Foreign Bodies

Treatment

If a foreign body enters the eye but is not embedded in the eyeball, attempt to remove it by irrigating the eye with a stream of water.

If irrigation does not remove the foreign body, carefully and gently attempt to lift out the material with a moistened cotton swab or cloth. Sometimes the foreign body will lodge underneath the upper eyelid. To examine under the upper lid, have the victim look downward as you grasp the eyelashes with your thumb and finger. Place the cotton end of a cotton-tipped applicator in the middle of the upper lid. Using the applicator as a fulcrum, pull the lid forward and upward, causing it to fold back over the applicator (inside out), exposing the undersurface of the lid (**Fig. 26a & b**). The foreign object can then be removed with the corner of a moistened cloth or another cotton swab.

After objects are removed from the eye, victims often report feeling as if something is still in their eye. This is usually caused by small scratches on the surface of the cornea. Treat the same as for a scratched eye (see "Scratched Eye [Corneal Abrasion]," page 42).

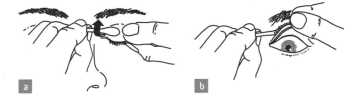

Fig. 26 *Everting the eyelid with a cotton-tipped applicator to locate a foreign body*

Weiss Advice

Eye Irrigation

Pour disinfected water into a sandwich or garbage bag and puncture the bottom of the bag with a safety pin. Squeeze the top of the bag firmly to create an irrigation stream, which can then be directed into the eye.

Eye Infections

Signs and Symptoms

Eye infections are characterized by red, itchy eye(s) with yellow or green discharge, crusted eyelashes, and swollen lids.

Treatment

Irrigate the eye with water. Antibiotic eyedrops can be prescribed by a physician. Tobramycin (Tobrex) drops applied to the eye every 2 to 3 hours while awake are an excellent choice.

Styes or Abscesses

Most bumps on the eyelid are styes.

Signs and Symptoms

A stye is an inflamed oil gland on the edge of the eyelid, where the lash meets the lid. It appears as a red, swollen bump that looks like a pimple. It is tender, especially to the touch.

Treatment

When a stye begins to develop, apply warm, moist compresses to the eyelid for 30 minutes four times a day until the stye either disappears or enlarges and comes to a head. If it comes to a head but does not drain spontaneously, seek medical attention. If the victim is more than 48 hours from medical care and the redness and/or swelling are progressing to include the cheek or forehead, carefully lance the stye with a scalpel or pin, followed by antibiotic therapy with dicloxacillin, erythromycin, or cephalexin.

Glaucoma

Glaucoma is a rise in pressure within the eye. If this happens suddenly (acute or narrow-angle glaucoma), blindness can result.

Signs and Symptoms

Symptoms include severe eye pain, blurred vision or halos around lights, clouding of the cornea, and redness of the white part of the eye. Nausea, vomiting, and headache can also occur.

Treatment

1. A glaucoma attack can sometimes be relieved with pilocarpine drops instilled into the eye, but often the victim needs surgery.
2. Acetazolamide (Diamox) may be administered in a dose of 250 mg twice a day.
3. Evacuate the victim immediately and as quickly as possible to an ophthalmologist.

Eye Floaters and Flashing Lights
(Vitreous Separation and Retinal Tears and Detachments)

Almost everyone gets occasional floaters in front of their eyes. These are small spots, lines, clouds, cobwebs, or veils that move about in your field of vision, especially when you move your eyes and when you are looking directly at a light background.

Eye floaters are caused by tiny opacities inside the vitreous, which is the gel that fills the inside of your eye. Sometimes the vitreous gel shrinks as it ages. In nearsighted (myopic) individuals, the vitreous gel may shrink more suddenly and begin to peel away from the retina. This is called a vitreous separation or detachment. A vitreous separation will cause floaters to appear, often suddenly. As the gel peels away from the retina, it tugs on it. This mechanical tugging can cause you to see light flashes, and could lead to a retinal tear.

Retinal tears can usually be treated with laser in the ophthalmologist's office. Left untreated, however, retinal tears can quickly lead to a retinal detachment which then requires major surgery. A retinal tear can lead to a retinal detachment, and permanent loss of vision within a day or less, so seek medical care as soon as possible if you develop new floaters.

When to Worry

Floaters

If you suddenly develop new floaters, flashing lights, or a defect in your field of vision (like a curtain over one part of your visual field), you should see an ophthalmologist at once to make sure you don't have either a retinal tear or a retinal detachment.

Weiss Advice

Relieving Eye Pain

Drops of tea squeezed from a cool, nonherbal tea bag may help to soothe the eye and relieve pain and redness.

EAR
Middle Ear Infection (Otitis Media)

Signs and Symptoms
Symptoms of middle ear infection include throbbing or stabbing pain in the ear, decreased or muffled hearing, and fever. Occasionally, a yellow discharge may drain from the ear.

Treatment
Treatment consists of an oral antibiotic (amoxicillin or trimethoprim/sulfamethoxazole [Septra DS]) for 10 days, along with a decongestant such as pseudoephedrine (Sudafed).

Swimmer's Ear (Otitis Externa)

Swimmer's ear is an infection of the outer ear caused by water and bacteria.

Signs and Symptoms
The first sign of swimmer's ear is usually itching and vague discomfort in the ear canal. Within a few to 24 hours, the ear can become red and extremely painful and drain yellowish fluid. Victims will have increased pain when you pull on the earlobe or push against the outer ear.

Treatment

Antibiotic eardrops containing polymyxin B sulfates and neomycin with hydrocortisone (Cortisporin Otic Suspension), should be placed into the outer ear canal four times a day for 4 to 5 days. Keep all water out of the ear for 2 to 3 weeks.

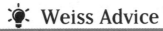 **Weiss Advice**

Treating Swimmer's Ear

If you don't have antibiotic eardrops, one part household vinegar diluted with four parts clean water or rubbing alcohol may be used as a substitute.

NOSE
Nosebleed

Treatment

Nosebleeds usually can be controlled by pinching the soft part of the nostrils together between your fingers and holding firmly for at least 15 to 20 minutes. If blood continues to drain down the back of the throat despite pinching the nostrils tightly, it indicates a posterior (back of the nose) bleed, which is a serious problem, because the victim can lose a significant amount of blood and it can interfere with their breathing. If the bleeding does not stop on its own after a few minutes, you may need to pack both the back and front of the nose (see Weiss Advice, pages 49 & 50). If the bleeding stops when you pinch the nostril, but resumes when you let go after 20 minutes of firm pressure, you may need to pack only the front of the nose.

☼ Weiss Advice

Packing the Front of the Nose

If bleeding cannot be controlled by pinching the nostrils together for a full 20 minutes, consider nasal packing (**Fig. 27a–c**).

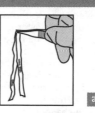

1. If available, insert into the nose a piece of cotton or gauze soaked with a blood vessel constrictor (e.g., Afrin or Neo-Synephrine nasal spray). Leave it in place for 5 minutes, and then remove it.

2. Cut a large gauze pad or soft cotton cloth into a thin continuous strip. Coat this with petroleum jelly or antibiotic ointment (**Fig. 27a**).

3. Gently pack the material into the nostril, using tweezers or a thin twig so that both ends of the packing material remain outside of the nasal cavity. Start the packing with the middle of the strip to keep the packing from going down the back of the throat. To completely pack the nasal cavity of an adult, you will need about 1 m (3 feet) of packing (**Fig. 27b**).

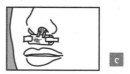

4. Secure the ends of the pack to the face with tape. (**Fig. 27c**).

5. Leave the pack in for 24 to 48 hours, then gently remove it. If bleeding starts again, repack the nostril.

Fig. 27 *Packing the front of the nose*

6. Packing the nose will block sinus drainage and predispose the victim to a sinus infection. Antibiotics such as Septra, Augmentin, Keflex, amoxicillin, or Zithromax should be taken until the packing is removed.

🔆 Weiss Advice

Packing the Back of the Nose

Bleeding from the back of the nose can be difficult to control and requires a posterior pack. A 5-mm (14–16 French) Foley catheter (something you may want to add to your first-aid kit) can be used to pack the back of the nose.

1. First, lubricate the catheter with either petroleum jelly or antibiotic ointment, then insert it through the nasal cavity to the back of the throat. (If the victim's mouth is open, you should be able to see the tip of the catheter in the throat behind the tongue.) Inflate the balloon of the catheter with 10 to 15 mL of air from a syringe.
2. Then gently draw the catheter out of the nose until resistance is met (**Fig. 28a & b**).
3. Secure the catheter firmly to the victim's forehead with several strips of tape.
4. Pack the front of the nose (as described on the previous page).

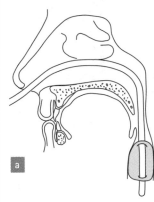
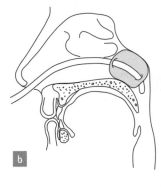

Fig. 28 *Packing the back of the nose*

DENTAL EMERGENCIES
Toothache

The common toothache is caused by inflammation of the dental pulp and is often associated with a cavity.

Signs and Symptoms

The pain may be severe and intermittent, and is made worse by hot or cold foods or liquids.

Treatment

1. If the offending cavity can be localized, a piece of cotton soaked with a topical anti-inflammatory agent such as eugenol (oil of cloves) can first be applied.
2. Place a temporary filling material, such as Cavit or zinc oxide and eugenol cement, into the cavity or lost filling site to protect the nerve.

☀ Weiss Advice

Replacing a Lost Filling

Melt some candle wax and allow it to cool until it is just soft and pliable. Place the wax into the cavity or lost filling site and smooth it out with your finger. Have the victim bite down to seat the wax in place. Remove any excess wax. Dental or orthodontic wax, often used to protect braces, is more pliable and works even better.

☀ Weiss Advice

Relieving Dental Pain and Bleeding

Bleeding and pain from the mouth can often be relieved by placing a moistened nonherbal tea bag onto the bleeding site or into the socket that is bleeding. Leave it in place for 5 to 10 minutes.

Dental Infections and Abscesses
Signs and Symptoms
Dental pain associated with swelling in the gumline at the base of the tooth might indicate a tooth infection or abscess. Tapping the offending tooth causes pain, but the tooth should not be sensitive to heat or cold. Dental infections occasionally spread beyond the tooth to the floor of the mouth, face, and neck. If this occurs, the victim may have difficulty opening the mouth, swallowing, or breathing, and fever and swelling of the face may develop.

Treatment
Make every effort to locate a dentist, as dental infections and abscesses can lead to serious illness and often require intravenous antibiotics, as well as extraction of the tooth or root canal therapy. Swelling of the face indicates a much more severe infection and can lead to a life-threatening condition. If a dentist cannot be reached, oral antibiotics (penicillin 500 mg, four times a day) should be started along with warm-water mouth rinses.

Displaced Tooth
If a tooth is knocked out, it may be salvageable if replaced within 30 to 60 minutes. A child's primary tooth (milk tooth) should not be placed back in the socket.

Treatment
Clean the debris off the tooth by rinsing gently (do not scrub!) with saline, milk, or disinfected water. Gently replace the tooth into the socket. The tooth should be handled only by the crown and not by the root. If the tooth cannot be replaced immediately, store it in a container with (in the following order of preference) tissue culture medium, saline, milk, or saliva.

Loose Tooth
Treatment
A tooth that becomes loosened, but not displaced, due to trauma should be repositioned with gentle, steady pressure. A soft diet should be maintained to avoid any further trauma until the tooth heals. The victim should see a dentist as soon as possible for definitive treatment.

CHEST INJURIES

Because wounds to the chest interfere with the ability to breathe, the victim requires immediate medical attention.

Broken Ribs

A forceful blow to the chest may break one or more ribs. Broken ribs are very painful and usually require pain medication and rest.

Signs and Symptoms

- Pain in the chest becomes worse with a deep breath.
- A crackling or rattling sensation or sound can occasionally be detected when touching the broken rib.
- Rib fractures usually occur along the side of the chest. Pushing on the breastbone (sternum) while the victim lies face up will produce pain at the fracture site rather than where you are pushing.

Treatment

Oral pain medication ibuprofin (Motrin) or acetaminophen with hydrocodone (Vicodin) will help reduce pain and make breathing easier. It takes about 2 weeks for pain to subside and 4 to 6 weeks for the rib to heal. Taping the chest over the fractured rib may provide added relief from pain.

When to Worry

Chest Injuries

One end of a broken rib can sometimes be displaced inward and puncture the lung, thus producing a pneumothorax (see "Collapsed Lung [Pneumothorax]," page 54). Rib fractures can also bruise the lung or predispose the victim to pneumonia. If a lower rib is fractured, it may injure the spleen or liver and cause severe bleeding. Multiple rib fractures can produce a flail chest (see "Flail Chest," page 54). Immediate evacuation to a medical facility is indicated if the victim has more than one rib fracture or develops shortness of breath, difficulty breathing, persistent cough, fever, abdominal pain, or dizziness or light-headedness upon standing.

Flail Chest

When three or more consecutive ribs on the same side of the chest are each broken in at least two places, a free-floating segment called a flail chest can result.

Signs and Symptoms

The flail segment will move opposite to the rest of the chest during breathing and make it hard for the victim to get enough air. The movement of broken ribs causes great pain, which further reduces the victim's ability to breathe. The underlying lung is usually bruised with a flail chest.

Treatment

1. Immediately evacuate the victim to a medical facility. A flail chest can be tolerated only for the first 24 to 48 hours, at which time the victim will usually need to be put on a respirator for breathing assistance.
2. Place a bulky pad of dressings, rolled-up extra clothing, or a small pillow gently over the site, or splint the victim's arm against the injury to stabilize the flail segment and relieve some of the pain. Whatever is used should be soft and lightweight. Use large strips of tape to hold the padding in place. Do not tape entirely around the chest, as this will restrict breathing efforts. The main function of this object is to make it less painful to breathe, not to stop movement of the chest or restrict breathing in any manner. Transport the victim lying faceup or on the injured side.
3. If the victim is severely short of breath and cannot get enough air, it may be necessary to assist with mouth-to-mouth rescue breathing. Time your breaths with those of the victim, and breathe gently to provide added air with each inspiration.

Collapsed Lung (Pneumothorax)

A collapsed lung (pneumothorax) occurs when air enters the chest cavity and compresses or collapses the lung. This can occur when a broken rib punctures the lung, an outside object such as a knife penetrates the chest, or even spontaneously when a weak point develops in the lung and permits air to leak into the chest cavity.

Signs and Symptoms
- Sharp chest pain, which may become worse with breathing
- Shortness of breath or difficulty breathing
- Reduced or absent breath sounds on the injured side

Treatment
Evacuate the patient immediately and monitor closely for the development of a tension pneumothorax (see "Tension Pneumothorax," below).

Tension Pneumothorax
A pneumothorax can progress to a life-threatening condition (a tension pneumothorax) if air continues to leak into the chest cavity. With each breath, air enters the space surrounding the lung, but it cannot escape with expiration. Pressure soon builds up, compressing the lung and heart, a condition that can eventually lead to death.

Signs and Symptoms
- Labored breathing
- Cyanosis (bluish skin discoloration)
- Signs of shock (weak, rapid pulse; rapid breathing; fear; pale and moist skin; confusion)
- Distended jugular (neck) veins
- Diminished or absent breath sounds on the injured side (Place your ear on the chest wall of the victim.)
- Bubbles of air felt or heard (a crackling sound) when touching the chest wall or neck

Treatment
If the situation is desperate and the victim is literally dying before your eyes, you can do only one thing to possibly save the life: you must relieve the pressure from inside the chest (pleural decompression) and allow the lung to re-expand. This procedure takes courage and

improvisation in the wilderness. *Pleural decompression should not be undertaken lightly and should be attempted only if the victim appears to be dying.* The possible complications include infection; profound bleeding from puncture of the heart, lung, or a major blood vessel; or even laceration of the liver or spleen.

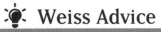 **Weiss Advice**

How to Perform Pleural Decompression

Caution: This technique should only be performed in the wilderness by a trained individual on a victim who would die if the procedure were not done.

1. Swab the entire chest with povidone-iodine or another antiseptic.
2. If sterile gloves are available, put them on after washing your hands.
3. If local anesthesia is available, inject it into the skin at the site to numb the area.
4. Insert into the chest a large-bore (14-gauge) intravenous catheter, needle, or any pointy, sharp object (not wider than a pencil) just above the third rib in the midclavicular line (approximately midway between the top of the shoulder and the nipple, in line with the nipple). If you hit the rib, move the needle or pointy object upward slightly until it passes over the top of the rib, thus avoiding the blood vessels that course along the bottom of every rib. A gush of air will signal that you have entered the correct space—do not push the object in any farther. This will convert the tension pneumothorax into an open pneumothorax.
5. Leave the object in place. Slit the finger portion of a rubber glove and cover the opening of the object with the slit glove to create a one-way flutter valve that allows air out but not in.
6. Anchor the object to the chest wall with tape so that it cannot be pulled out or forced farther into the chest.
7. Monitor the victim closely, and if signs of tension redevelop, repeat the procedure.

Open (Sucking) Chest Wound

If an object such as a bullet or knife enters the chest, a wound that opens into the lung can develop. Each time the victim breathes, a sucking sound often can be heard as air passes in and out through the hole.

Signs and Symptoms
- Painful and difficult breathing
- A sucking sound each time the victim breathes
- Bubbles visible at the wound site when the victim exhales
- Bubbles of air that can be felt and heard (crackling sounds) when touching the chest wall near the injury
- A tension pneumothorax (see "Tension Pneumothorax," page 55)

Treatment
1. Seal the opening immediately with any airtight substance and cover it with a 10 x 10-cm (4 x 4-inch) gauze pad, then tape it on three sides. (Taping three edges produces a flutter valve effect. When the victim inhales, the free edge will seal against the skin. As the victim exhales, the free edge will allow air in the chest cavity to escape.)
2. If an object is stuck in the chest, do not remove it. Place airtight material next to the skin around it, and stabilize it with bulky dressings or pads. Several layers of dressings, clothing, or handkerchiefs placed on the sides of the object will help stabilize it.

A victim with an open chest wound below the nipple line may also have an injury to an abdominal organ such as the spleen or liver (see "Abdominal (Belly) Injuries," page 58).

☀ Weiss Advice

Dressing an Open Chest Wound

An airtight dressing can be improvised from a 10 x 10-cm (4 x 4-inch) gauze pad impregnated with petroleum jelly, honey, or antibiotic ointment. Plastic wrap or clean plastic will also work. Tape the dressing in place on three sides only.

ABDOMINAL (BELLY) INJURIES

Abdominal organs are either solid or hollow. When solid organs such as the spleen or liver are injured, they bleed internally. Hollow organs can rupture and drain their contents into the abdominal and pelvic cavities, producing a painful and serious inflammatory reaction and infection.

Organ	Type	Location
Liver	Solid	RUQ
Stomach	Hollow	LUQ
Spleen	Solid	LUQ
Pancreas	Solid	LUQ
Small and large intestines	Hollow	All quadrants
Kidneys	Solid	Flanks

RIGHT UPPER QUADRANT (RUQ)

LEFT UPPER QUADRANT (LUQ)

RIGHT LOWER QUADRANT (RLQ)

LEFT LOWER QUADRANT (LLQ)

Penetrating Injuries
(See "Gunshot Wounds and Arrow Injuries," page 60.)

Blunt Abdominal Injuries
A blow to the belly can result in internal organ injuries and bleeding, even though nothing penetrates the skin. Examine the abdomen by pressing on all four quadrants sequentially and gently with the tips of your fingers. Push slowly and observe for pain, muscle spasms, or rigidity. Normal abdomens are soft and not painful when touched.

Signs and Symptoms
- Signs of shock (see "Shock," page 32)
- Pain that is at first mild and then becomes severe
- Distention (bloating) of the abdomen
- Pain or rigidity (tightness or hardness) of the belly muscles when pressing in on the abdomen
- Pain referred to the left or right shoulder tip, which may indicate a ruptured spleen
- Nausea or repetitive vomiting
- Bloody urination
- Pain in the abdomen on movement
- Fever

Treatment
1. Immediately evacuate the victim to a medical facility.
2. Anticipate and treat for shock.
3. Do not allow the victim to eat. If the victim is not vomiting, offer small sips of water.

GUNSHOT WOUNDS AND ARROW INJURIES
Gunshot Wounds

Injuries caused by guns differ in severity and type according to velocity of the bullet, power of the gun, whether fragmentation occurs, presence of powder burns, and type of tissue struck.

Signs and Symptoms

A gunshot wound may cause severe internal damage and bleeding that are not readily visible or apparent. Although the entrance or exit wound may appear small, the damage inside the body may be great. Any victim who has suffered a gunshot wound should be brought to a medical facility immediately, no matter how minor the external appearance.

Treatment

1. Follow the basic principles of resuscitation, including airway, breathing, circulation, control of bleeding, immobilization of any broken extremities, wound care, and stabilization of the victim for transport (see "Life-Threatening Emergencies," page 22).
2. Remove the weapon from the vicinity where you are giving medical care. It may be wise also to remove the ammunition and open the firing chamber.
3. Provide immediate relief of a tension pneumothorax with pleural decompression (see "Tension Pneumothorax," page 55).
4. Treat any sucking chest wound with petrolatum-impregnated gauze (see "Open [Sucking] Chest Wound," page 57).
5. Control external bleeding with direct pressure and compression wraps.
6. Treat for shock and hypothermia (see "Shock," page 32).
7. Monitor the neurovascular status of an extremity wound.
8. Keep the extremity elevated to minimize swelling.
9. Be aware that the path of the bullet cannot be determined by connecting the entrance and exit wounds.
10. For powder burns, remove as much of the powder residue as possible with a scrub brush, because the powder will tattoo the skin if left in place.
11. Expect internal bleeding (see When to Worry, page 62).

Arrow Injuries

Arrowheads are designed to inflict injury by cutting tissue and blood vessels.

Signs and Symptoms

Arrow injuries can cause bleeding and shock.

Treatment

1. Follow the same treatment recommendations as for a firearm injury.
2. Stabilize the victim for transport, leaving any embedded arrow in place during transport if possible. Cut the shaft of the arrow and leave about 10 cm (4 inches) protruding from the wound to make transport easier (see "Do Not Remove Embedded Foreign Objects," below).
3. Fix the portion of the arrow that remains in the wound with a stack of gauze pads or with cloth and tape.
4. Transfer the victim as quickly as possible to a medical care facility for removal of the arrow under controlled conditions.

Do Not Remove Embedded Foreign Objects

If a foreign object (such as a knife, tree limb, or arrow) becomes deeply embedded (impaled) in the body, do not attempt to remove it. Because the internal portion may be up against or in a vital organ and acting as a plug, thus preventing further bleeding, any attempt to remove the object may cause further bleeding and injury. This is particularly true with a hunting (broadhead) arrow. Instead, pad and bandage the wound around the object and secure it in place with tape. The portion of the object that is sticking out of the wound may be carefully cut shorter to facilitate splinting. Transport the victim immediately thereafter.

⟲ When to Worry

Internal Bleeding

If bleeding is internal (inside the body), such as from an injured spleen or liver, bleeding ulcer, broken bone, or torn internal blood vessel, the victim may suffer from shock. The symptoms of internal bleeding—rapid heartbeat, low blood pressure, shortness of breath, weakness, pale skin color, cool and clammy skin, and confusion—are the same as those of external bleeding except that no blood will be visible. The belly may feel firm to the touch and look distended, and the victim may feel abdominal pain. Blood may be present in the vomit, urine, or stool. Because it is difficult to predict the rate and severity of internal bleeding, the victim should be immediately transported to professional medical attention.

KNEE INJURIES
Knee Sprain

Twisting, rotating, or falling in an awkward position can produce a sprain injury to one of the major ligaments that supports the knee. The collateral ligaments support the sides of the knee, while the anterior and posterior cruciate ligaments support and limit motion in the forward and backward directions.

Signs and Symptoms

The victim may note an audible crack or a pop at the time of injury, followed by immediate pain that soon turns into a dull ache. The ache may subside after a while, and the knee will swell and feel as though it's going to give way when you put weight on it or turn to the side.

Knee sprains are divided into three degrees of severity based on the amount of ligament that is torn:

1. *First-degree sprains* produce pain but no instability when the knee is stressed, indicating that only a few ligament fibers are torn. Treatment is initially RICES: rest, ice, compression, elevation, and stabilization (see "RICES," page 66) and later physical therapy. Walking can usually be resumed with little or no additional support.

2. *Second-degree sprains* produce pain and slight instability when the knee is stressed, indicating that about half the ligament fibers are torn. Treatment is the same as for a first-degree sprain, but recovery takes longer and surgery may eventually be required. The victim should wear a supportive knee immobilizer while walking (**Fig. 29**).

3. *Third-degree sprains* produce significant instability and indicate a completely torn ligament. Initiate treatment with RICES and prohibit walking without a supportive knee immobilizer in place. Even with a third-degree tear, many victims will still be able to walk out of the wilderness with some additional support.

Treatment

If after applying an improvised knee immobilizer (see Weiss Advice, below), the knee still feels unstable and prone to buckling with weight, the victim should be evacuated without walking.

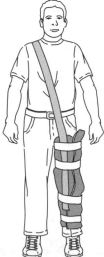

Fig. 29
Duct-tape suspenders supporting an improvised knee immobilizer

☀ Weiss Advice
Knee Immobilizer

A knee immobilizer (knee splint) can be improvised from an Ensolite or Therm-a-Rest pad, life jacket, newspaper, firm blanket, tent poles, or internal pack frame stays and clothing held together with tape or bandannas. The immobilizer should be cylindrical and extend from mid-thigh to mid-calf. If possible, cut out a circular hole for the kneecap. Duct tape can be used to fashion suspenders to prevent the knee immobilizer from slipping downward while walking (**Fig. 29**).

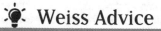

Patellofemoral Syndrome

This common overuse syndrome produces a dull, aching pain under the kneecap or in the center of the knee. The pain is aggravated by climbing or descending hills and by sitting for long periods with the knees bent.

Signs and Symptoms

The knee may be swollen, and crackling sounds can often be heard when the knee is flexed and straightened.

Treatment

Treatment is rest, ice, and anti-inflammatory medication such as ibuprofen (Motrin) 400 mg three times a day with meals. A patella tendon band placed around the leg, below the kneecap, may help prevent pain during walking (see Weiss Advice, below). Use of two trekking or ski poles while hiking will help absorb impact on the knees.

☀ Weiss Advice

Patella Tendon Band

To improvise a patella tendon band, roll a bandanna or triangular bandage tightly along its long axis. Wrap this around the leg just below the kneecap and tie it securely.

Torn Meniscus (Cartilage)

Menisci are pieces of cartilage that act as shock absorbers for the knee and rest between the thigh and shin bones. Partial and total tears of a meniscus often occur at the same time that ligaments are torn.

Signs and Symptoms

Pain, localized to one side of the knee joint and made worse by walking, is the most common symptom. Clicking or locking of the knee may be present. Occasionally, the joint can become locked in a partially flexed and painful position, and the victim will not be able to move the knee.

Treatment

1. Treatment is rest, ice, and ibuprofen (Motrin) 400 mg three times a day with meals.
2. If the knee feels unstable, wrap a protective immobilizer around it (see **Fig. 29**, page 63).
3. If the victim has a locked knee, attempt to unlock it by positioning the victim with the leg hanging over the edge of a table or flat surface with the knee in approximately 90 degrees of flexion. After a period of relaxation, apply in-line traction to the leg with inward and outward rotation in an attempt to unlock the joint. Pain medications and muscle relaxers (if available) may facilitate this.

SPRAINS

A sprain is the stretching or tearing of ligaments that attach one bone to another. Ligaments are sprained when a joint is twisted or stretched beyond its normal range of motion. Most sprains occur in the ankle and knee.

Signs and Symptoms

Symptoms include tenderness at the site, swelling, bruising, and pain with movement. Because these symptoms are also present with a fracture, it may be difficult to differentiate between the two.

Treatment

First aid for sprains is primarily damage control and summarized by RICES (see "RICES," page 66). RICES should be maintained for the first 72 hours after any injury. Too often this treatment is prematurely discontinued after only a few hours.

Administer a nonsteroidal anti-inflammatory drug (NSAID) such as ibuprofen (Motrin) 400–600 mg three times a day with food to reduce both pain and inflammation.

As soon as possible, seek medical evaluation to determine the need for X-rays to check for a fracture.

RICES FOR SPRAINS AND STRAINS

REST: Resting takes the stress off the injured joint and prevents further damage.

ICE: Ice reduces swelling and eases pain. For ice or cold therapy to be effective, it must be applied early and for up to 20 minutes at least three to four times a day, followed by compression bandaging. If a compression wrap is not applied after ice therapy, the joint will swell as soon as the ice is removed.

COMPRESSION: Compression wraps prevent swelling and provide some support. A compression wrap can be made by placing some padding (socks, gloves, pieces of Ensolite pad) over the sprained joint and then wrapping it with an elastic bandage. Begin the wrap toward the end of the extremity and move upward. For example, with an ankle sprain, start from the toes and move up the foot and over the ankle with the wrap. The wrap should be comfortably tight. If the victim experiences numbness, tingling, or increased pain, the compression wrap may be too tight and should be loosened.

ELEVATION: Elevate the injured joint above the level of the heart as much as possible to reduce swelling.

STABILIZATION: Tape or splint the injured part to prevent further injury (see Weiss Advice, page 68).

Ankle Sprain
Sprained ankles are common backcountry injuries. Most commonly, the ligaments on the outside of the joint are injured when the foot is rolled inward (inverted) while walking or jumping on an uneven surface.

Treatment
1. First aid begins with RICES. If the victim cannot bear weight at all, splint the foot and ankle (see **Fig. 47**, page 93) and get assistance out of the backcountry.
2. If the victim can still walk, tape the ankle for support with an open-basket cross-weave stirrup pattern to prevent further injury (**Fig. 30a & b**).
   a. Apply an anchor strip halfway around the lower leg about 15 cm

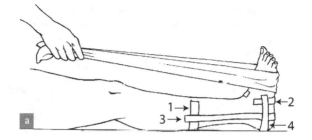

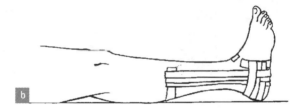

The numbers indicate the order in which the pieces of tape are applied.

Fig. 30 *Sprained ankle taping using a cross-weave stirrup pattern*

(6 inches) above the "bumps" in the ankle. Leave a gap of 4 cm (1.5 inches) between the ends of the tape to allow for swelling.

b. An additional anchor strip can be applied at the instep of the foot. Leave a 4-cm (1.5 inches) gap between the tape ends.

c. Apply the first of five stirrup strips. Beginning on the inside of the upper anchor, wrap a piece of tape down the inside of the leg, over the inside bump, across the bottom of the foot, up the outside part of the leg, and over the outside bump, ending at the outer part of the upper anchor.

d. Apply the first of six interconnecting horseshoe strips. Start on the anchor on the inside of the foot and wrap below the inside bump, around the heel, and below the outside bump, ending on the anchor on the outer part of the foot.

e. Repeat steps c and d. Remember to overlap the tape by one-half its width. These interlocking strips should provide excellent support when walking. After applying these vertical and horizontal strips, there should be a 2.5- to 5-cm (1- to 2-inch) gap on the top of the foot and ankle, which will allow for any swelling.

f. On both sides, secure the tape ends with two vertical strips of tape running from the foot anchor to the calf anchor.

☀ Weiss Advice

Ankle Support with a C-Splint

Wrap a C-Splint (**Fig. 31a–c**) around the foot and ankle, with the shoe in place, and secure it with tape. This will help stabilize the joint while walking. You may need to stop periodically to tighten or rewrap the splint.

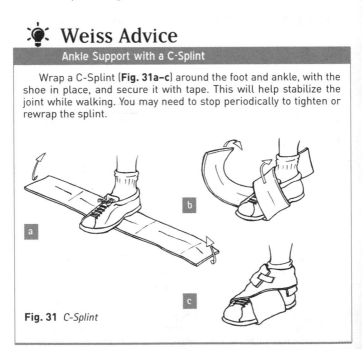

Fig. 31 *C-Splint*

STRAINS

A strain is an injury to a muscle or a tendon. (Tendons connect muscle to bone.) Strains often result from overexertion or from lifting and pulling a heavy object without good body mechanics. Strains can sometimes be disabling, especially in the back. Symptoms and treatment are the same as for sprains.

Muscle spasms often accompany a strain injury and can be very painful. Muscle relaxers such as diazepam (Valium), cyclobenzaprine (Flexeril), or carisoprodol (Soma) may be helpful in relieving spasms, but they also produce drowsiness and poor coordination.

As a rule of thumb, the following times are required for initial healing of the musculoskeletal system:

- Muscles: 6–8 weeks
- Bones: 6–12 weeks
- Tendons and ligaments: 12–36 weeks (some ligaments may take 12 months or longer to heal)

Strained or Ruptured Achilles Tendon

Running or walking uphill with a heavy load on the back can injure the Achilles tendon, which attaches the calf muscles to the heel. The tendon can even rupture completely while running or jumping, in which case it pulls away from the bone or snaps in half.

Signs and Symptoms

A ruptured Achilles tendon feels like someone has stabbed the back of the ankle with a sharp object, making it impossible to bear weight. The victim will often hear a snap as the tendon ruptures.

Treatment

If the tendon is not completely torn or ruptured, **RICES** is the best treatment. Gently stretch the tendon to keep it flexible, and gradually put weight on the foot, then walk as the pain allows. A ruptured Achilles tendon will make walking impossible. The ankle should be splinted (see **Fig. 47**, page 93) and the victim evacuated. Surgery is needed to repair the torn tendon.

BACK PAIN

Back pain ranks among the top ten most common ailments of backpackers. The lower part of the back, the lumbar spine, holds most of the weight of the body, and therefore is most likely to give you problems. Preventing a back injury is a lot easier than trying to recover from one. While on the trail, several things can be done to lessen the chances of back injury.

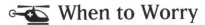 # When to Worry

Back Pain

If back pain is severe and not made worse with movement or a change in position, it may be due to some other internal problem, such as an aortic aneurysm or kidney infection, that can cause pain to radiate to the back. In such cases, it is important to see a physician at once. Shooting pains, tingling down the leg, loss of sensation in an arm or leg, problems with bowel or bladder function, and leg or foot weakness are also reasons to seek medical attention immediately.

Back Strain

Prevention

- Stretch before lifting a pack, especially in the morning when muscles are cold and stiff.
- When putting on a heavy pack, keep the back straight and in a neutral position. Slide the pack onto one thigh and slip one shoulder into a loosened shoulder strap. Roll the pack onto the back while using the legs, not the back and arms, to lift up.
- When lifting, always keep objects close to the body.
- Adjust the pack so as much weight as possible is on the hip belt, instead of the shoulder straps.
- Use a walking stick for added balance and support.

Although back pain may be a symptom of a more serious condition, it is often due to strained muscles.

Treatment

If possible, it is helpful to rest on the back with a pillow under the knees or lie on the side with a pillow between the legs for 1 to 2 days before resuming gentle and graded activity. Extended bed rest and inactivity can actually weaken the back and delay recovery. Most people with sudden back pain will recover completely within 2 to 4 weeks.

Other treatments include the following:

1. Anti-inflammatory medication such as ibuprofen (Motrin) 600 mg three times a day (with meals) for 5 to 7 days
2. Application of cold compresses
3. Gentle massage
4. Muscle relaxers to relieve muscle spasms diazepam (Valium), cyclobenzaprine (Flexeril), or carisoprodol (Soma)

Kidney Stones

Kidney stones are hard deposits that develop in the urinary tract and produce extreme pain that is often felt in the back. These stones range in size from a grain of sand to a marble. Kidney stones are three times more common in men than in women and typically develop during middle age. Dehydration and a diet high in protein or calcium are predisposing factors.

Signs and Symptoms

Sudden onset of very severe pain, usually starting in the flank area, or one side of the back and radiating to the abdomen or groin, is typical of kidney stone pain. The victim often rolls from side to side in an effort to find a more comfortable position. With appendicitis or other abdominal infections, the victim usually lies still because movement will increase the pain. Other symptoms may include nausea, vomiting, an urge to urinate, and blood in the urine.

Treatment

1. Consumption of plenty of fluids—at least 4 L (1 gallon) a day—may help to flush out the stone and prevent new stones from forming.
2. Pain medication should be administered to the victim. An excellent medication for kidney stone pain is ibuprofen (Motrin) 600 mg three times a day or another nonsteroidal anti-inflammatory drug.
3. Most kidney stones will eventually pass on their own. Occasionally, kidney stones can lead to infection and damage to the kidney.

Kidney Infections
A kidney infection (pyelonephritis) will often produce back pain and can be mistaken for a back injury (see "Urinary Tract Infections," page 126).

FRACTURES
A fracture is any break or crack in a bone. An open, or compound, fracture occurs when the overlying skin at the fracture site has been punctured or cut. This can happen when a sharp bone end protrudes through the skin or from a direct blow that breaks the skin as it fractures the bone. The bone may or may not be visible in the wound. A closed fracture is one in which there is no wound on the skin anywhere near the fracture site. A closed fracture can become an open fracture if it is not handled carefully.

Open fractures are more likely than closed fractures to produce significant blood loss. They also increase the possibility that the bone will become contaminated or infected due to being exposed to the environment. An infected bone is very difficult to treat and may cause long-term problems.

How to Tell if a Bone Is Fractured
It may be difficult to differentiate a fractured bone from a sprained ligament or bruised muscle. When in doubt, splint the extremity and assume it is fractured until you can obtain an X-ray.

Signs of a Possible Fracture
- Deformity (The limb appears to be in an unnatural position. Compare the injured limb with the uninjured limb on the opposite side. Look for differences in length, angle, or rotation.)
- Pain and tenderness over a specific point (point tenderness)
- Inability to use the extremity (For example, someone who twists an ankle and is unable to bear weight should be suspected of having a broken ankle rather than a sprained ankle.)
- Rapid swelling and bruising (black-and-blue discoloration)
- Crepitus (A grating or grinding sensation can sometimes be felt and heard when touching or moving a fractured limb.)
- Motion where no joint exists

Treatment: General Guidelines

1. Inspect the site of injury for any deformity, angulation, or damage to the skin. Instead of removing the victim's clothing, cut away the clothing at the fracture site with blunt-tipped scissors. This will prevent excess movement and better protect the victim from the environment.
2. Stop any bleeding with direct pressure.
3. Check the circulation below the fracture site by feeling for pulses and inspecting the skin for abnormal color changes. Pallor (paleness), bluish discoloration, or a colder hand or foot compared with the noninjured side may indicate a damaged blood vessel. Without circulation, a limb can survive only for about 6 to 8 hours. Check sensation by using a safety pin to determine if the sharp sensation is felt equally on both extremities.
4. Because of the force necessary to break a bone, carefully examine any person with a fracture for other injuries.
5. Unless the victim's life is in immediate danger, splint all fractures before moving. Splinting prevents movement of the broken bones, which avoids additional injury to bones, muscles, nerves, and blood vessels. It also reduces pain, prevents a closed fracture from becoming open, and makes evacuating the victim easier.

Treatment of Open Fractures

Irrigate the wound with large amounts of sterile saline or disinfected water to remove any obvious dirt, then cover it with a sterile dressing. After thoroughly cleansing the wound and bone, try to realign (straighten) the extremity to its normal position to facilitate splinting (see "Splinting," page 74). Don't worry if the bone is pushed back under the skin, as this is better than leaving it exposed.

Realignment of an Open Fracture

1. After thorough irrigation of the wound and while someone else holds counter-traction on the limb above the fracture, pull gently on the limb below the fracture site in a direction that straightens it.
2. While continuing to hold traction, immediately apply a splint to prevent further motion and damage.
3. Cover the wound with a sterile dressing and bandage.

Splinting

In general, a splint should be long enough to incorporate the joints above and below the fracture. The splint should be rigid and well padded. The splint should immobilize the fractured part in a position of function. Functional position means that the leg is almost straight with slight flexion at the knee (place a rolled-up towel behind the knee), the ankle and elbow are bent at 90 degrees, the wrist is straight or slightly extended, and the fingers are flexed in a curve as if one were attempting to hold a can of soda or a baseball.

- Remove all jewelry, such as watches, bracelets, and rings, before applying the splint.
- Use plenty of padding, especially at the bony protrusions of the wrist, elbow, ankle, and knees.
- Secure the splint in place with strips of clothing, belts, pieces of rope, webbing, pack straps, elastic bandages, or duct tape.
- Fashion the splint on the uninjured body part first, then transfer it to the injured area to minimize discomfort.
- Elevate the injured body part as much as possible after splinting to minimize swelling.
- Always check the circulation after applying a splint or doing any manipulation. Check the pulse in the foot or wrist, skin color, and temperature often to ensure that swelling inside the splint has not cut off circulation.
- Administer pain medicine to the victim.

Realignment of a Closed Fracture

In general, straightening a fractured limb is not advised, unless circulation to the extremity is impaired or gross deformity prevents splinting and transportation. Realignment is easier if it is done soon after the injury occurs and before swelling and pain make doing so more difficult (see **Fig. 32**).

1. While someone holds counter-traction on the limb above the fracture, pull gently on the limb below the fracture site in a direction that straightens it. Discontinue the maneuver if the patient complains of a dramatic increase in pain.
2. After the limb has been straightened, immediately apply a splint

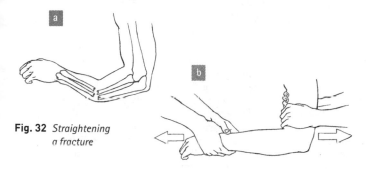

Fig. 32 *Straightening a fracture*

before releasing traction. If alignment cannot be achieved, splint the extremity as it is.

3. After any manipulation, recheck to see whether circulation has been restored or improved.

TREATMENT OF SPECIFIC FRACTURES
Neck and Spine Fracture

Fractures of the neck and spine can damage the spinal cord and lead to permanent paralysis. Any accident that places excessive force or pressure on the head, neck, or back, such as a fall, head injury, or diving accident, can also result in a fracture of the spine.

The decision to initiate and to maintain spine immobilization in the wilderness has significant ramifications. An otherwise walking victim would require a potentially expensive and arduous rescue. The added delay could worsen other injuries and predispose the victim and the rest of the party to hypothermia or other environmental hazards. Although in general it is always better to err on the side of being overprotective, everyone with a bump or cut on the head does not need to have the spine immobilized.

If a spine injury is suspected, the rescuer should immobilize the head, neck, and trunk to prevent any movement. If the victim is lying in a dangerous location and must be moved quickly, the victim's head and neck should be held firmly by one rescuer's hands, while as many people as available place their arms under the victim from either side. The rescuer at the head says, "Ready, go," and with everyone lifting simultaneously, the victim is lifted as a unit and moved to a safer location. After the victim is moved, one rescuer should continue to hold the head firmly with two hands until the spine is completely immobilized.

If the neck lies at an angle to the body, it should be straightened with gentle in-line traction. A second rescuer should then place a cervical collar around the neck to provide some stability. Cervical collars alone do not provide adequate immobilization. After a collar is placed around the neck, plastic bags, stuff sacks or socks filled with sand or dirt, or rolled-up towels and clothing should be placed on either side of the head and neck and secured to the head with tape or straps to prevent any side-to-side movement. The rest of the body should then be secured to a flat board to prevent any movement.

If the victim needs to be turned onto their side because of vomiting, maintain spine precautions by logrolling the victim (see **Fig. 15**, page 27).

When to Worry

Spinal Injury

Suspect a spinal injury, and initiate and maintain spine immobilization after trauma that involves the head, neck, or back, under these circumstances:

- The victim is unconscious.
- The victim feels pain in the back of the neck or the middle of the back, or experiences discomfort when those areas are touched.
- The victim reports numbness, tingling, or diminished sensation in any part of an arm or leg.
- The victim exhibits weakness or inability to move the arms, legs, hands, or feet.
- A victim has an altered level of consciousness (see "Head Injuries," page 33) or is under the influence of drugs or alcohol. (Under these circumstances, the exam may not be reliable.)
- A victim has another very painful injury, such as a femur or pelvic fracture, dislocated shoulder, or broken rib, that may distract him from noticing pain in the neck.

☀ Weiss Advice

Improvised Cervical Collars

A cervical collar can be improvised by using a C-Splint, sleeping pad, newspaper, backpack hip belt, fanny pack, sleeping pad, life jacket, or clothing.

C-Splint Cervical Collar
Create a bend in the C-Splint approximately 15 cm (6 inches) from the end of the splint. This bend will form the front support, which holds the chin. Place the front support underneath the chin and wrap the remainder of the splint around the neck. Create side supports

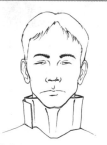

C-Splint cervical collar

by squeezing together the slack in the splint to form flares under each ear. Finally, squeeze the back of the splint in a similar manner to create a back support, and secure the whole thing with tape.

Sleeping Pad Collar
Fold the pad lengthwise into thirds, then center it over the back of the victim's neck. Wrap the pad around the neck, then under the chin, and secure it in place with tape. If the pad is not long enough, tape or tie on extensions. Blankets, beach towels, or even a rolled plastic tarp can be used in a similar fashion.

Padded Hip Belt Collar
A padded hip belt taken from a large internal- or external-frame backpack can sometimes be modified, after removal, to function as a cervical collar. If the belt is too long, overlap the ends and secure them with duct tape.

Clothing Collar
Any bulky item of clothing can be used. Before placing it on the neck, wrap a wide elastic-type bandage around the entire item to compress the material and to make it more rigid and supportive.

Jaw Fracture

Signs and Symptoms

A fracture of the mandible (jawbone) should be suspected if the victim has pain and swelling at the site or is unable to open or close the mouth normally, or the teeth do not fit together in a normal fashion.

Treatment

Apply ice to the site to reduce swelling and pain. Maintain a liquid diet until the victim reaches the hospital.

Facial Fracture

Fractures of the nose and cheekbones are the most common fractures of the face. These occur from direct blows to the face and can be associated with other head injuries such as a concussion of the brain or eye or dental injuries.

Signs and Symptoms

- The victim may feel tenderness when the cheekbones or bones around the eyes are touched.
- The skin exhibits swelling and black-and-blue discoloration.
- Grasp the upper teeth between your thumb and forefinger and gently rock the teeth back and forth. Abnormal movement of the upper face when you do this indicates a fracture.
- The victim may have double vision, especially when looking upward.
- The fractured side of the face may feel numb.
- The nose may appear swollen and deformed, and there may be bleeding from the nostrils.

Treatment

1. Elevate the victim's head and apply ice to reduce swelling.
2. See treatment for nosebleeds (see "Nosebleed," page 48).
3. Administer pain medication (see Appendix D).
4. Evacuate the victim to a medical facility.

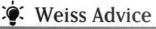

Weiss Advice

Making a Shoulder Sling with Safety Pins

If the victim is wearing a long-sleeved shirt or jacket, pin the injured arm to the chest portion of the garment with two safety pins. If the victim is wearing a short-sleeved shirt, fold the bottom of the shirt up and over the injured arm to create a pouch. Pin the pouch to the sleeve and chest section of the shirt to immobilize the arm.

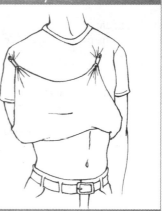

Fig. 33 *Shoulder immobilizer using the victim's own shirt and two safety pins*

Collarbone (Clavicle) Fracture

A collarbone fracture most likely occurs from a fall directly onto the shoulder.

Signs and Symptoms

The victim will usually hold the arm against the chest wall for support and to prevent motion of the broken bone. The collarbone will be tender to the touch, and a lump or swelling may be present at the site.

Treatment

Splint the arm against the chest with a sling and swath, or with safety pins (**Fig. 33**).

Shoulder and Upper Arm (Humerus) Fracture

Signs and Symptoms

There is usually pain and tenderness when the site is touched and inability to use the arm are typical indications of a humerus fracture.

Unlike dislocations of the shoulder, victims with a fracture can still bring the injured arm in tightly and comfortably against the chest and can touch the opposite shoulder with the hand of the injured arm.

Treatment
Upper arm fractures should be immobilized with a well-padded splint that extends from the armpit down the inner part of the arm, around the elbow, and back up the outside of the arm to the shoulder. After splinting, secure the arm against the body using a sling and swath, or safety pins (**Fig. 33**). Flex the elbow less than 90 degrees to avoid pinching off any blood vessels.

Elbow, Forearm, or Wrist Fracture
Such fractures usually occur after a fall on an outstretched hand.

Signs and Symptoms
A broken wrist sometimes has a deformity, which makes it look like an upside-down fork.

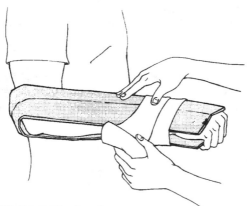

Fig. 34 *C-Splint for elbow, forearm, or wrist fracture*

Treatment

1. For an obvious deformity where circulation has been cut off to the hand (no pulse at the wrist, the hand is turning blue and cold compared with the uninjured hand), apply firm traction to straighten the deformity.
2. Include the elbow and hand in a splint for a wrist, forearm, or elbow fracture. Apply a well-padded, U-shaped splint that extends from the hand to the elbow on both sides and wraps around the elbow like a sandwich. Bend the elbow at 90 degrees; keep the wrist as straight as possible; and arrange the hand in a position of function with the fingers curled around something soft, such as a rolled-up glove, sock, or bandage (**Fig. 34**).
3. After splinting, secure the arm against the body for added support.

☀ Weiss Advice

The C-Splint for Arms

The C-Splint, a versatile and lightweight padded aluminum splint, is excellent for splinting upper extremity fractures. It goes from being flexible to rigid when bent into a U-shape down its long axis. The C-Splint can be used for splinting arms in almost any position. Place the blue side of the splint, slightly thicker and softer than the orange side, against the skin.

Hand and Finger Fracture

Fractures of the hands and fingers usually result from bending of the bone, such as when someone's finger is pulled back or when a closed fist is driven into a solid object.

Signs and Symptoms

Pain and swelling will be evident at the site of the fracture, and deformity may be noticeable.

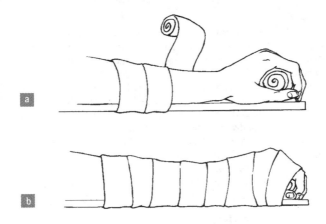

Fig. 35 *Splint for hand fractures, with fingers curled around a roll or bandage*

Treatment

After removing any jewelry, place a rolled pair of socks or an elastic bandage in the palm to keep the fingers curled in a grabbing position (position of function) and secure this in place with an elastic or gauze bandage (**Fig. 35**). Keep the tips of the fingers uncovered in order to check circulation.

Splint a broken finger by buddy-taping the injured finger to an adjacent uninjured finger (**Fig. 36**). Elevate hand injuries to minimize swelling.

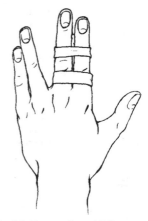

Fig. 36 *Finger splint, with fingers buddy-taped*

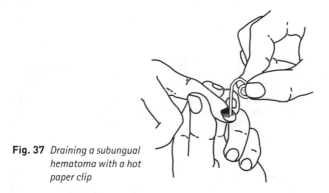

Fig. 37 *Draining a subungual hematoma with a hot paper clip*

Blood Under a Nail (Subungual Hematoma)

A subungual hematoma is a collection of blood underneath a fingernail or toenail that causes severe throbbing pain. The condition often results from a traumatic injury, such as slamming a finger in a door, hitting the end of the finger with an object like a hammer, or during sports such as climbing.

Signs and Symptoms

- There is throbbing pain under the nail.
- The nail develops black or blue discoloration directly underneath it.

Treatment

1. Subungual hematomas are treated by drilling a hole through the nail into the hematoma to relieve the pressure (**Fig. 37**).
2. First, immerse the finger in cold or ice water to help numb the nail bed.
3. Heat the end of an opened paper clip or similar object in an open flame and then apply the hot tip to the nail. Use steady pressure until resistance is no longer felt and the blood drains out.
4. Gently squeeze the tip of the finger to facilitate drainage of the blood.
5. Apply a dressing to the finger.

Rib Fracture
(See "Chest Injuries," page 53).

Pelvis Fracture
Pelvic-ring fractures are devastating injuries, often accompanied by extensive internal bleeding that frequently can be fatal. In addition to losing large amounts of blood into the pelvis from broken bones and torn blood vessels, the victim with a pelvic fracture often has other major internal injuries and bleeding. The victim can go into shock and bleed to death internally without any sign of external bleeding. Organs such as the bladder or intestines also may be damaged.

Signs and Symptoms
There may be pain in the pelvis, hip joint, or lower back, and inability to bear weight. Pressing or squeezing gently on the pelvis at the belt-line will produce pain. If the broken pelvis is unstable, you may feel the movement of the bones when you compress the pelvis. If you find an unstable pelvis during your assessment, don't do any further exams of the pelvis. Pressing or squeezing the pelvis further can dislodge internal blood clots and cause more bleeding. If the bladder or urethra is damaged, blood may travel to the tip of the penis or into the urine, or the victim may be unable to urinate.

Treatment
Stabilization and compression of the broken pelvis with a pelvic sling or binder will help control bleeding and may save the victim's life. It's a technique that works even for the worst type of pelvic fractures, known as open-book fractures because the pelvic ring has sprung open like the pages of a book. Compression "closes the book," reduces pain, slows bleeding, and promotes clot formation as the patient is transported to an emergency department.

In the backcountry, you can use an inflatable sleeping pad (**Fig. 38**), or clothes, sheets, sleeping bags, pads, or a tent fly to improvise a pelvic sling (**Fig. 39a–c**). First, remove any objects from the victim's pockets and any belt the victim is wearing so that pressure of the sling doesn't cause additional pain by pressing items against the pelvis. Then slide a

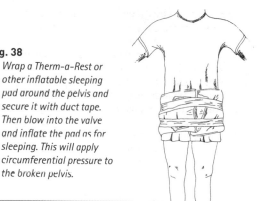

Fig. 38

Wrap a Therm-a-Rest or other inflatable sleeping pad around the pelvis and secure it with duct tape. Then blow into the valve and inflate the pad as for sleeping. This will apply circumferential pressure to the broken pelvis.

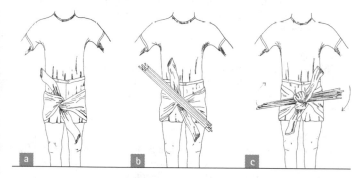

Fig. 39

   a *Slide an article of clothing or sheet or tent fly under the victim's pelvis and center it under the bony prominences at the outer part of the hips. Cross this over the front of the pelvis and tie it together with an overhand knot.*

   b *Place tent poles, a stick, or similar object on the knot and tie another overhand knot.*

   c *Twist the poles or stick until the pelvic sling becomes tight.*

sheet, jacket, sleeping pad, or other improvised sling under the victim's buttocks and center it under the bony prominences at the outer part of the upper thighs or hips (greater trochanters/symphysis pubis). Cross the object over the front of the pelvis and tighten the sling by pulling both ends and securing them with a knot, clamp, or duct tape. Tighten the sling so that it is snug. If you use an inflatable sleeping pad, inflate it after securing to increase the pressure exerted on the pelvis.

Place padding between the legs and gently tie the legs together to further stabilize the fracture in a position that is most comfortable for the victim. Treat for shock, but do not elevate the legs. Transport the victim if possible on a well-padded but firm surface, or better yet, arrange for a helicopter evacuation.

Thigh Bone (Femur) Fracture

A broken femur can produce severe blood loss and lead to shock. When the femur breaks, the thigh muscles spasm, pulling the thigh into a more spherical shape, which allows a greater amount of blood to escape into the surrounding tissues.

Signs and Symptoms

The broken bone ends will overlap and dig into the muscle, causing additional injury, extreme pain, and further blood loss. Often, the broken leg will appear shortened and the foot may be rotated outward, away from the other leg.

Treatment

The best splint for a femur fracture is one that produces traction to stretch the muscles back to their normal length (see Weiss Advice, page 87). This will significantly reduce blood loss, muscle spasms, and pain and will facilitate evacuation. First, apply traction with your hands by holding the victim's foot and pulling the leg back into normal alignment. Try to pull the injured leg out to its normal length, using the uninjured leg as a guide. Once you have started pulling traction, do not release it. If it's just you and the victim, create a traction splint first, then pull and maintain traction with the device.

☀ Weiss Advice

Traction Splint

A variety of techniques are available for improvising a traction splint with limited materials in the backcountry. An improvised traction splint has six components:

■ Ankle hitch
■ Upper thigh (crotch) hitch
■ Rigid support that is longer than the leg
■ Method for securing the two hitches to the rigid support
■ Method for producing traction (trucker's hitch)
■ Padding

WARNING: Before applying an improvised splint to the victim, test your creation on an uninjured member of your party, or at least on the uninjured leg of the victim.

1. Apply an ankle hitch. It is best to leave the shoe on the victim's foot and apply the hitch over it. Cut out the toe of the shoe so you can periodically check the circulation in the foot.

Double runner stirrup. Fold two long, narrow, and strong pieces of material (webbing, triangular bandages or bandannas folded into cravats, pieces of rope, or even shoelaces) into loops and lay one over and one behind the ankle, making sure the ends of each loop are facing in opposite directions (**Fig. 40**). Pull the ends through the loop on both sides. The hitch

Fig. 40 *Double runner stirrup ankle hitch*

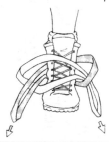

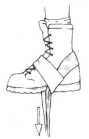

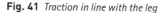

Fig. 41 *Traction in line with the leg*

should fit snugly and flat against the ankle. Adjust the two pieces of material so that the ends are centered under the arch of the shoe and the traction is in line with the leg (**Fig. 41**). The foot should be at a 90-degree angle with the ankle.

S-configuration hitch. This type of hitch is preferred if the victim also has an injury to his foot or ankle, because traction is pulled from the victim's calf instead of the ankle. Lay a long piece of webbing or other similar material over the upper part of the ankle (lower calf) in an S-shaped configuration. Wrap both ends of the webbing behind the ankle and up through the loop on the other side. Pull the ends down on either side of the arch of the foot to tighten the hitch and tie an overhand knot (**Fig. 42**).

Buck's traction. For extended transports, this system is more comfortable but must be checked periodically for slippage. Wrap duct tape around a piece of Ensolite or another sleeping pad to create a stirrup (**Fig. 43**). Secure the entire unit to the lower leg with an elastic or other improvised bandage. This system greatly increases the surface area over which traction is applied and decreases the potential for painful pressure points and compression of blood vessels leading to the foot.

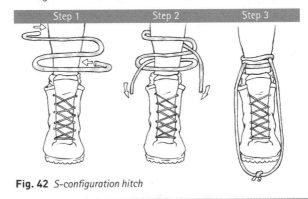

Fig. 42 *S-configuration hitch*

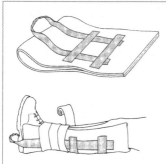

Fig. 43 *Buck's traction*

2. Apply the upper thigh hitch. Tightly wrap a rolled-up jacket or other material (belt, webbing, fanny pack, or pack straps) around the upper part of the thigh and tie an overhand knot. Climbers can use a climbing harness, while paddlers can use an inverted life jacket worn like a diaper. Regardless of the material used, make sure to pad the crotch and inner thigh.

3. Apply a rigid support to the outside of the injured leg. Secure it between the two hitches. Place a rigid, straight object that is at least a foot longer than the leg against the outside of the leg and secure it to the upper thigh hitch with tape or strapping material. You can use, for example, one or two ski poles lashed together with duct tape, a ski, tent poles, a canoe or kayak paddle, or a straight tree branch.

4. Attach the ankle hitch to the rigid support. A blanket pin or bent tent stake can be placed in the end of a tent pole to provide an anchor for the traction system. A Prusik knot (**Fig. 44**) can be used as an attachment point on almost any straight object.

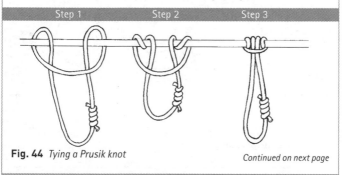

Step 1   Step 2   Step 3

Fig. 44 *Tying a Prusik knot*

Continued on next page

Continued from previous page

5. Apply traction. The amount of traction required will vary with the individual. A stopping point for pulling traction is when the injured leg appears to be its normal length again (compare it with the uninjured leg) or when the victim is more comfortable. Use a trucker's hitch to gain mechanical advantage when pulling traction (**Fig. 45**). After applying traction, check the circulation and sensation in the foot every 30 minutes. If the pulse is lost or diminished with traction, or if the foot turns blue or cold, reduce the amount of traction in the splint until the color and pulse return.

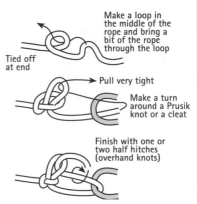

Make a loop in the middle of the rope and bring a bit of the rope through the loop

Tied off at end

Pull very tight

Make a turn around a Prusik knot or a cleat

Finish with one or two half hitches (overhand knots)

Fig. 45 *Trucker's hitch*

6. Apply padding. Pad the foot, ankle, and leg at all points where they come into contact with the splint and hitches. Secure the entire splint firmly to the leg (**Fig. 46**).

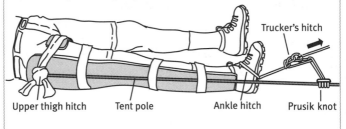

Upper thigh hitch   Tent pole   Ankle hitch   Prusik knot

Trucker's hitch

Fig. 46 *Completed femoral traction splint with Prusik knot used as an anchor for pulling traction*

Knee Fracture

Fractures of the knee either involve the kneecap (patella), the lower end of the femur, or the upper end of the tibia or fibula.

Signs and Symptoms

- A fracture of the kneecap will produce severe pain and tenderness directly over the kneecap and inability to bend or straighten the knee without dramatically increasing the pain.
- There will be swelling around the knee.
- A fracture of the upper tibia will produce pain just below the kneecap and inability to bend or straighten the knee without increasing the pain. The victim will not be able to walk without significant pain.

Treatment

Fractures around the knee should be splinted from the hip to the ankle with a cylinder splint (see Weiss Advice, page 63). You can use a life jacket or rolled-up sleeping pad. Individuals with fractures near the knee should not be allowed to walk without crutches.

Lower-Leg (Tibia and Fibula) Fracture

The tibia can fracture from a direct blow or from a twisting force to the bone, as seen in ski injuries. The principal danger associated with a tibia fracture is the development of a compartment syndrome, in which bleeding and swelling in the calf lead to increased pressure in the calf. If the pressure gets high enough, vital structures, such as nerves, blood vessels, and muscle, are squeezed, leading to permanent damage.

Signs and Symptoms

- Deformity of the limb at the fracture site
- Crepitus (grinding sound) when leg is moved
- Tenderness at the fracture site
- Immediate swelling

A victim with a tibia fracture will not be able to bear weight. Some victims with an isolated fibula fracture can still walk on the injured leg—but with pain.

Treatment

If necessary, apply gentle traction to straighten any deformity that exists in the leg and maintain the traction while another person applies a splint. For lower-leg fractures, apply a splint that encompasses the leg from the knee to the ankle. A U-shaped splint running from the inner thigh above the knee around the bottom of the foot and up the outside of the leg back to the knee, with adequate padding, is an excellent splint. After splinting, elevate the leg to reduce swelling. Check the circulation and sensation in the foot every 30 minutes. Numbness and tingling in the foot, severe pain produced when the rescuer moves the victim's toes, or loss of pulse in the foot are potential signs of a compartment syndrome. If any of these symptoms occur, loosen the splint, elevate the leg higher, and speed up the evacuation if possible.

Ankle and Foot Fracture

The ends of the tibia and fibula overlap the smaller ankle bones slightly, producing bumps on either side of the ankle. When the ankle is twisted, the outer bump (the lateral malleolus) sometimes cracks. This is the most common ankle fracture.

Signs and Symptoms

It can be difficult to differentiate a broken ankle bone from a severe ligament sprain without X-rays. Both injuries can produce swelling, pain, and black-and-blue discoloration. If the victim is unable to bear weight, or if gentle pressure directly on the upper part of the bony prominences on the inside or outside of the ankle produces severe pain, treat the injury as a fracture.

Treatment

Apply a well-padded splint that begins halfway down the calf and extends around the bottom of the foot and back up the other side, encompassing the ankle like a sandwich. Splint the ankle so that the

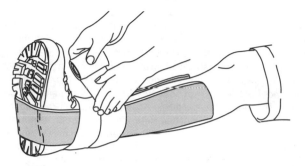

Fig. 47 *U-shaped splint for immobilizing a broken ankle or one of the bones in the lower leg*

foot rests at a 90-degree angle to the leg (**Fig 47**). Leave the boot or shoe in place, but remove the tongue so that you can periodically check circulation and sensation. Keep the foot elevated above the level of the heart as much as possible.

Foot and Toe Fracture

Bones in the feet can be fractured by direct trauma, such as a heavy object dropped onto the foot. Fractures of the toes usually occur when the victim stubs or catches a toe on an obstacle.

Signs and Symptoms

- Swelling and pain at the fracture site
- Possible black-and-blue discoloration
- Noticeable deformity if fracture displaced

Treatment

Splint a fractured toe by buddy-taping it to an adjacent toe with small pieces of tape. Place cotton or gauze material between the toes to prevent rubbing and chafing. Victims with a fractured foot or toe may still be able to walk out of the backcountry under their own power with a walking stick and the foot supported in a protective and well-padded shoe.

DISLOCATIONS

A dislocation is the displacement or separation of bones in a joint from their normal position. Dislocations often damage the supporting structures of the joint and tear ligaments. Sometimes a bone under strain may "pop" out of position (subluxation) and pop back in again. This will be painful but does not require reduction (relocation or returning the bone to normal position). A subluxation is treated as a sprain injury. Dislocations are most common in the shoulders, elbows, fingers, and kneecap (patella).

The reduction of a dislocation (returning the bone to its normal position) by nonphysicians is controversial in wilderness medicine. There are many good reasons for reducing a dislocation in the backcountry, especially when rapid transport to a hospital is not possible:

- Reduction is easier soon after injury, before swelling and muscle spasm develop.
- Reduction relieves pain.
- Early reduction reduces the risk of further injury to blood vessels, nerves, and muscles. Blood vessels can become trapped, stretched, or even compressed during a dislocation, which leads to loss of blood flow to the limb if reduction is not performed.
- It is easier to splint the extremity and evacuate the victim after reduction.

Even if a fracture accompanies the dislocation, the first step in treatment is to attempt to reduce the dislocation (although a fracture may sometimes prevent reduction of the dislocation).

If you are unable to reduce the dislocation immediately, administering pain relievers and muscle relaxers, and waiting at least 20 minutes for them to take effect, may make the procedure go more easily. Use steady, constant traction when attempting a reduction. After any dislocation is reduced, the extremity should be splinted in the same manner as for a fracture. If a dislocation can't be reduced, splint the extremity in the most comfortable position for the victim.

Shoulder Dislocation

Shoulder dislocations are common in kayakers and skiers because paddles and ski poles place added force on the joint. For a shoulder dislocation to occur, the arm is usually pulled away from the body, rotated outward, and extended backward. This can occur when a kayaker high braces or attempts to roll the kayak. The arm gets yanked out of its socket and lodges in front of the joint.

Signs and Symptoms

Victims are usually in severe pain and aware that something is out of joint. The shoulder may look squared off, lacking the normal rounded contour. The victim will usually hold the arm away from the body with the uninjured arm and be unable to bring it in tightly into the chest (**Fig. 48**). If the victim can bring the arm across the body in a normal position for splinting and touch the opposite shoulder with the hand, then you should assume a shoulder dislocation is not the problem.

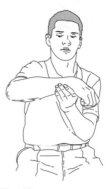

Fig. 48

The victim with a dislocated shoulder holds the arm up and away from the body and is unable to bring the arm in against the chest, as one would for splinting.

Treatment

Before attempting to reduce the shoulder, check the pulse in the wrist (radial pulse) and the circulation (temperature, color, and capillary refill) in the hand. Check the nerve function by asking the victim to move the wrist up and down and move all the fingers. Test for sensation to touch or pinprick.

Many good techniques are available for reducing a shoulder dislocation. In the backcountry, the key is to do it quickly, before the muscles spasm.

WEISS TECHNIQUE FOR SHOULDER REDUCTION (STANDING)

Have the victim bend over at the waist while you support the chest and allow the arm to hang toward the ground. Support as much of the victim's weight as possible to allow him to relax. With your other hand, grab the victim's wrist and turn the arm slowly so that the palm faces forward. Then apply steady downward traction and very slowly bring the

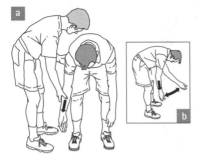

Fig. 49 *One-person Weiss technique (standing) for reducing a dislocated shoulder*

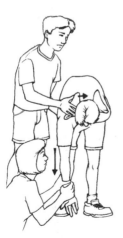

Fig. 50 *Two-person Weiss technique (standing) for reducing a dislocated shoulder*

arm forward toward the head (**Fig. 49**). Avoid jerky movements. You may need to hold traction for a few minutes before the bone pops back into the shoulder socket.

If two rescuers are available, one should support the victim at the chest and provide counter-traction while the other pulls downward on the arm. The person supporting the chest also can use the thumb of the other hand to push the scapula (shoulder blade) inward toward the backbone (**Fig. 50**). This scapular manipulation maneuver helps position the socket so the arm can slip back in more easily. You can usually notice a clunk and shift of the arm as it returns to the joint, combined with a sigh of relief from the victim.

ONE PERSON SHOULDER REDUCTION (SITTING)

While the victim is sitting, grab the forearm close to the elbow with both of your hands. With the victim's elbow bent at 90 degrees, apply steady downward traction on the arm by pulling on the forearm. After about a minute of sustained traction, slowly raise the entire arm upward, until reduction is complete. Gingerly rotating the forearm outward while pulling traction may facilitate reduction. Another rescuer can provide counter-traction from behind the victim while scapular manipulation is being performed, as described above (**Fig. 51**).

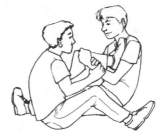

SHOULDER REDUCTION WITH VICTIM SUPINE

Fig. 51 *One-rescuer (sitting) technique for reducing a dislocated shoulder*

If the standing or sitting shoulder reduction technique is unsuccessful, the next preferred technique is to have the victim lie flat on his back with the dislocated arm held straight out from the side of the body. The arm should be flexed at the elbow and the forearm held in a vertical position. A loop of clothing or sheet that has been tied around the rescuer's waist should be slipped over the arm and down to the

Fig. 52 *Shoulder reduction technique with victim supine and second rescuer*

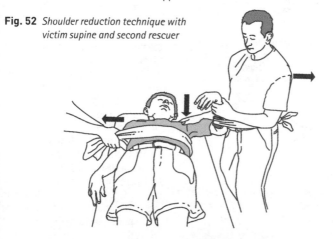

SHOULDER SPICA TO SUPPORT THE ARM AND SHOULDER

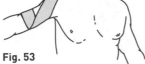

Fig. 53

Begin by encircling the upper arm with wide (6-inch is best) elastic bandage and continue upward to the armpit. Continue the wrap around the shoulder.

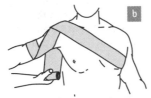

Wrap the bandage across the chest and under the opposite shoulder, through the armpit, and around the back to the injured shoulder.

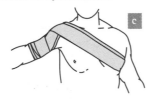

Repeat the pattern as the length of the bandage allows and finish on the upper arm.

elbow. After padding the elbow, the rescuer can apply traction by leaning backward. A second rescuer must hold counter traction on the injured victim with a loop of clothing around the chest, to prevent the body from moving when traction is applied to the arm (**Fig. 52**).

After the shoulder is reduced, recheck the victim's circulation, sensation, and ability to move the fingers and wrist. Immobilize the arm with a sling and swath bandage, or with safety pins (see **Fig. 33**, page 79)

After a shoulder dislocation is reduced, or if there is a shoulder strain or sprain injury and the victim will need to use the arm to facilitate an exit from the wilderness (such as a kayaker who needs to paddle down the river to a takeout), a shoulder spica can be used to support and help protect the injured shoulder. The spica should be applied after a shoulder dislocation is reduced, if the victim must continue to use the involved arm (**Fig. 53a–c**).

WARNING: If you cannot reduce a dislocated shoulder after two attempts, or if the reduction maneuver produces a dramatic increase in pain, abort the attempt and splint the arm in the most

comfortable position for the victim. This usually requires placing
a pillow or rolled blanket under
the armpit, between the arm and
chest wall.

Elbow Dislocation
Signs and Symptoms
When the elbow is dislocated,
there will be a deformity at the
joint when compared with the
uninjured side, and movement of
the elbow will be very limited and
painful. Check for a pulse in the
wrist and determine if the victim
can move the fingers and wrist.

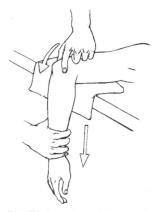

Fig. 54 *Reducing a dislocated elbow*

Treatment
Elbow dislocations require a great deal of traction and may be impossible to reduce in the backcountry. If you are unable to reduce the dislocation, splint the arm in the most comfortable position for the victim. To
attempt reduction, have the victim lie face down with the elbow bent at
90 degrees over the padded edge of a table or ledge. Pull downward on
the wrist while another rescuer pulls upward on the upper arm. Rocking
the forearm back and forth gently may help the reduction (**Fig. 54**). After
any reduction attempt, recheck the pulse in the wrist and circulation to
the fingers.

After reduction, splint the elbow as though it were a fracture (see
"Elbow, Forearm, or Wrist Fracture," page 80).

Finger Dislocation
Signs and Symptoms
Someone with a dislocated finger will be unable to move the dislocated joint and a deformity will be obvious. Do not attempt to reduce a
dislocation at the base of the index finger. Splint this injury in a position
of comfort and seek medical attention.

Treatment

Pull on the tip of the finger with one hand, while pushing the base of the dislocated finger with the other hand (**Fig. 55**). After reduction, buddy-tape the reduced finger to an adjacent finger (see **Fig. 36,** page 82).

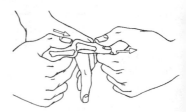

Fig. 55 *Reducing a dislocated finger*

Hip Dislocation

Signs and Symptoms

In most hip dislocations, the femur is pushed out and back, dislodging behind the hip socket. The victim's leg is rotated inward, and the hip and knee are both flexed. The victim will be in a great deal of pain and unable to move or straighten the injured leg.

Treatment

Two people and a lot of force are required to reduce a pelvic dislocation. Place the victim on his back with the knee and hip both flexed at 90 degrees. One rescuer will hold the victim flat on the ground by pushing down with his hands on both sides of the victim's hips. The other rescuer straddles the victim's calf, locks hands behind the victim's knee, and applies steady traction in an upward direction (**Fig. 56**).

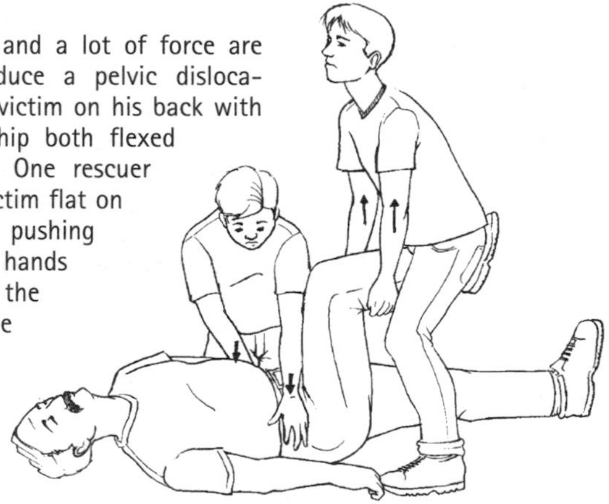

Fig. 56
Reducing a dislocated hip

Reducing a hip is often difficult and requires a great deal of pro-longed pulling to overcome the powerful leg muscles. Once reduced, splint the injured leg to the uninjured leg and transport the victim to a medical facility. If reduction is unsuccessful, splint the leg in the most comfortable position for the victim and ar-range evacuation.

Kneecap Dislocation
Dislocation of the kneecap (patella) usually occurs from a twisting injury while the knee is extended.

Signs and Symptoms
The kneecap is displaced to the outer part of the knee, resulting in an obvious deformity and pain. The knee is usually flexed, and the victim is unable to move it.

Treatment
A patella dislocation can usually be reduced by pushing the kneecap back toward the inside of the knee with the thumbs, while gently straightening the leg (**Fig. 57**). The kneecap will pop back into place, and the victim should experience immediate pain relief. If the maneuver is very painful or not easily accomplished, do not continue with the attempt. After

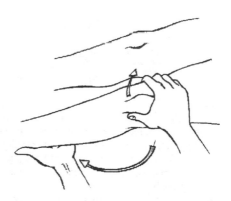

Fig. 57 *Reducing a kneecap dislocation*

the kneecap is repositioned, the victim should be able to walk with an improvised knee immobilizer (see Weiss Advice, page 63). If you're unable to reduce the dislocated patella, splint the knee in a position of comfort and evacuate the victim.

Knee Dislocation

Do not confuse this devastating injury with a dislocation of the knee-cap. A total knee dislocation results in the disruption of all of the ligaments of the knee and a very unstable joint. Often the knee will reduce itself spontaneously. If the knee is still deformed, gently reposition and straighten it by applying gentle traction to the lower leg. Evacuate the victim immediately to the nearest medical facility. A major artery in the leg is often torn or damaged during dislocation of the knee and, if not repaired within 6 to 8 hours, amputation of the leg may be necessary.

Ankle Dislocation

Sometimes a severe ankle fracture can also be dislocated. Apply gentle traction to the foot and ankle until the deformity has been corrected and the ankle is better aligned. Splint the ankle as you would for a fracture (see "Ankle and Foot Fracture," page 92).

WOUNDS: CUTS AND ABRASIONS

A wound can be anything from a small skin abrasion to a large cut (laceration). Effective wound management is not difficult to achieve, and it comes in handy both in the backcountry and at home. It can often save you a costly and lengthy trip to the emergency room.

Bleeding

Almost all bleeding can be stopped by applying direct pressure to the wound. Use whatever clean material is available to hold pressure on the bleeding site, then, as time allows, use sterile gauze from a first-aid kit. The idea is not to soak up blood with a big wad of bandage but, rather, to apply firm pressure directly on the bleeding site. If direct pressure does not stop the bleeding, examine the wound to make sure you are holding pressure on the correct spot before putting more bandages on top of those already in place. It might be necessary to hold pressure for up to 30 minutes to prevent further bleeding. If you need to free up your hands, create a pressure dressing by wrapping an elastic bandage tightly around a stack of 10 x 10-cm (4 x 4-inch) gauze pads placed over the wound.

If bleeding from an extremity cannot be stopped by direct pressure, and the victim is in danger of bleeding to death, apply a tourniquet. (A tourniquet is any band applied so tightly around an arm or leg that all blood flow beyond the band is cut off. See "How to Apply a Tourniquet," page 20.) If the tourniquet is left on for more than 4 hours, everything beyond the tourniquet will die, and that part of the arm or leg may require amputation.

Never apply direct pressure to a bleeding neck wound, because it can interfere with breathing. Instead, carefully pinch the wound closed. Never apply direct pressure to the eye, either, because that could cause permanent damage.

When bleeding cannot be controlled with direct pressure, QuikClot Sport hemostatic agent and QuikClot Emergency Dressings are useful products to apply to a bleeding wound. QuikClot Sport, an over-the-counter product, contains zeolite, a naturally occurring mineral that has been preloaded with moisture to eliminate the heat buildup that was present in the first generation of QuikClot products. QuikClot Sport's zeolite beads are contained in an easy-to-apply mesh pouch to be placed directly into the bleeding wound. QuikClot's third-generation products, available by prescription only, contain kaolin, a naturally occurring, inert mineral, and are available in gauze dressings. When either zeolite or kaolin comes into contact with blood in and around a wound, it assimilates the smaller water molecules found in the blood and activates and promotes blood clotting. With either product, once the dressing or mesh pouch is applied, direct pressure must be maintained for it to be effective.

Celox granules are another product that can help stop bleeding. When poured into a wound, the granules mix with blood and form a gel-like clot. To apply Celox, pour the granules from a sterilized, sealed packet into the wound, and then hold them in place with a gauze dressing. Apply a compression bandage by wrapping an elastic wrap bandage over the gauze and around the bleeding site.

Anytime you deal with blood, it's vitally important to wear barrier gloves to protect yourself from blood-borne pathogens, such as the hepatitis and HIV. Even latex gloves can leak, so make sure to wash your hands or wipe them with an antimicrobial towelette after removing gloves. Dispose of bloody gloves and bandage materials by securing them in a waterproof bag.

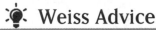 **Weiss Advice**

Stopping the Bleeding

Oxymetazoline (Afrin) and Phenylephrine (Neo-Synephrine) nasal sprays contain a medication that constricts (shrinks) blood vessels and may help stop wound bleeding. Simply moisten a 10 x 10 cm (4 x 4-inch) piece of gauze with the solution, then pack the gauze into the wound. A moistened, nonherbal tea bag may also help to control bleeding in the mouth. The tannic acid in tea acts as a blood-vessel constrictor and can even help relieve pain.

Cleaning a Wound

The moment skin is broken, bacteria begin to multiply inside a wound, and any blood or damaged tissue left behind will create a feeding ground for hungry germs. The goal of wound cleansing, therefore, is to rid the wound of as much bacteria, dirt, and damaged tissue as possible.

The best cleansing method is to use a 10 to 15 mL syringe with an 18- or 19-gauge catheter tip attached to the end to create a high-pressure irrigation stream (see "How to Irrigate a Wound," page 105). Using the syringe like a squirt gun creates an ideal pressure, forceful enough to flush out germs and debris without harming tissues.

Disinfected water is ideal for irrigating wounds. Water can be quickly disinfected by adding 10 mL (2 teaspoons) of 10% povidone-iodine (Betadine) solution to 0.5 L (1 pint) of backcountry water and allowing it to sit for 5 minutes. If the water is particularly dirty, pour it through a coffee filter, bandanna, or paper towel before disinfecting.

Do not pour hydrogen peroxide into wounds; it is damaging to tissue and can delay healing. Even full-strength 10% povidone-iodine (Betadine) solution is toxic to delicate skin tissues and should not be poured directly into a wound unless diluted first.

How to Irrigate a Wound

Draw disinfected water into the syringe and attach an 18-gauge catheter tip. Hold the syringe so the catheter tip is just above the wound and perpendicular to the skin surface. Push down forcefully on the plunger while prying open the edges of the wound with your gloved fingers, then squirt the solution into the wound. Be careful to avoid getting

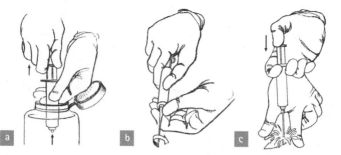

Fig. 58 *Wound irrigation*

splashed by the solution as it hits the skin (put on sunglasses or goggles to help protect your eyes from the spray). Repeat this procedure until you have irrigated the wound with at least 500 mL of solution. The more you use the better (**Fig. 58a–c**).

Inspect the irrigated wound for any residual particles of dirt or dried blood and, if present, carefully pick them out with clean tweezers. This is crucial because even one or two particles of dirt left in a wound will increase the likelihood of infection. Control any renewed bleeding by direct pressure.

☀ Weiss Advice

Wound Irrigation with a Plastic Bag and Safety Pin

Fill a plastic sandwich or garbage bag with disinfected water and puncture the bottom of the bag with a safety pin or pointy knife. Hold the bag just above the wound and squeeze the top firmly to begin irrigating.

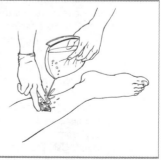

Wound Closure

Many cuts can be closed safely in the backcountry. Time is a critical factor, however, and the longer you delay closure, the more likely it is that the wound will become infected after being closed. The golden period for closing most wounds is within 8 hours after the injury occurs. If you wait longer, bacteria multiply inside the wound to a dangerous level and swelling progresses, interfering with the body's defense system. Wounds on the face or scalp can be closed up to 24 hours later because these areas are more resistant to infection.

Some wounds always carry a high risk of infection, regardless of when they are closed. Examples are wounds inflicted by animal or human bites, puncture wounds, deep wounds on the hands or feet, and those that contain a great deal of crushed or damaged tissue.

Most high-risk wounds, and those that have aged beyond the golden period, are best left open and packed with 10 x 10-cm (4 x 4-inch) gauze dressings moistened with saline solution or disinfected water. Cover the packed wound with a bandage, then splint the extremity. Administer antibiotics, if available. Change the packing at least once a day, and obtain professional medical care as soon as possible.

Otherwise, the preferred way to close a cut in the backcountry is with wound closure tape strips or butterfly bandages. Wound closure strips are better, because they are stronger, longer, stickier, and more porous than butterfly bandages.

Closing a Wound with Wound Closure Strips

1. Use your scissors to clip off hair near the wound so the tape will adhere better. Hair farther from the wound edge can be shaved. Avoid shaving hair right next to the wound edge as it abrades the skin and increases the potential for infection.
2. Apply a thin layer of tincture of benzoin or other topical skin adhesive, evenly along both sides of the wound, being careful to avoid getting the solution into the wound (it stings). Benzoin's stickiness will help keep the tape in place (**Fig. 59a**).
3. After the benzoin dries (about 30 seconds), remove a wound closure strip from its backing (**Fig. 59b**) and place it on one side of the wound. Use the other end of the strip as a handle to pull the wound closed (**Fig. 59c**). Try not to squeeze the wound edges

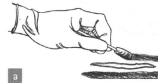

Fig. 59

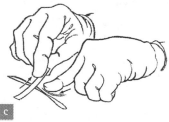

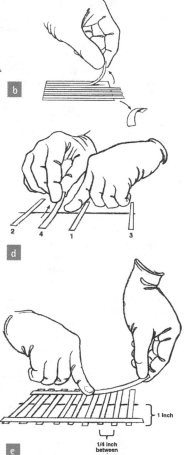

tightly together; they should just touch. Attach the other end of the strip to the skin to keep the wound closed.

4. Overlap the wound edge with the wound closure strip by about 2.5 cm (1 inch) on each side. Apply more tape as needed, with a gap of about 1 cm (0.5 inch) between each strip (**Fig. 59d**).

5. Place additional wound closure strips or pieces of tape crosswise (perpendicular to the other strips) over the ends of the existing strips to keep the ends of the strips from curling up (**Fig. 59e**).

6. Leave the strips in place 7 to 10 days.

🔅 Weiss Advice

Improvised Wound Closure Strips

Wound closure strip can be improvised from duct tape or other adhesive tape. Cut 0.5-cm (.25-inch) strips, then puncture tiny holes along the length of the tape with a safety pin to prevent fluid from building up under the tape. If you're without tape, you can even glue strips of cloth or nylon from your clothes, pack, or tent to the skin with superglue. Place a drop of glue on the material, and hold it on the skin until it dries. Use the other end to the pull the wound closed, then glue the strip onto the skin on the other side of the wound. Avoid getting any glue into the wound. The glue is generally safe on intact skin but should not be used on the face. Expect the strip to fall off after 2 or 3 days. If you are still in the backcountry then, reapply more strips with fresh glue.

Gluing a Wound Closed with Dermabond

2-octyl cyanoacrylate (Dermabond) is a topical skin adhesive for repairing skin lacerations. It is ideal for backcountry use because it precludes the need for topical anesthesia, is easy to use, doesn't require any needles, and takes up a lot less room in a backpack than a conventional suture kit. (Ask your physician to supply you with some for your wilderness outings.) When applied to the skin surface, Dermabond will keep wound edges stuck together for 3 to 4 days, and it peels off without leaving evidence of its presence. Do not substitute Krazy Glue or superglue for Dermabond, because they may cause injury to broken skin (see **Fig. 60**, page 109)

1. Irrigate the wound with copious amounts of disinfected water.
2. Control any bleeding with direct pressure (the glue will not hold well when it is applied to a bleeding wound).
3. Tissue glue is applied only to the outside surface of the wound to bridge over the edges; do not apply it directly into an open wound.
4. Gently squeeze the two wound edges together with your fingers so that the edges are straight, just touching each other, and lie together evenly. Be sure that the wound edges are matched correctly. Hold gauze against downstream areas to catch any

drippings as you apply the glue (**Fig. 60**).

5. While you hold the edges together, have an assistant paint the tissue glue over the joined wound edges, using a very light brushing motion of the applicator tip (**Fig. 60a**). Avoid excessive pressure of the applicator on the tissue because this could separate the skin edges and allow glue into the wound.

6. Apply multiple thin layers (at least three) of glue, allowing it to dry between applications (about 2 minutes).

7. If the wound is large and difficult to approximate with your fingers, first apply wound closure strips to close the wound edges (see "Closing a Wound with Wound Closure Strips," page 106), then glue between the strips (**Fig. 60b**). Next, remove one strip at a time and glue the skin where the strip had been.

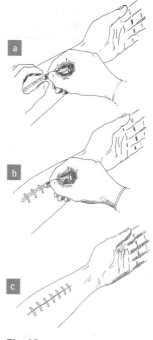

Fig. 60
Gluing a wound closed

8. Remove glue from unwanted surfaces with acetone, or loosen it from skin with petroleum jelly. (Do not use petroleum-based ointments and salves, including antibiotic ointments, on the wound after gluing, since these substances can weaken the glue and cause the wound to reopen.)

9. After the wound has been glued shut, apply or reapply wound closure strips to back up your closure (**Fig. 60c**).

Large, gaping cuts and wounds that are under tension or that cross a joint are difficult to tape or glue closed and may require suturing. In these instances, obtain professional medical care as soon as possible.

Scalp Lacerations

Scalp lacerations can often be closed by tying the victim's hair together (see Weiss Advice, page 37).

Dressing the Wound
The best initial dressing is one that won't stick to the wound. Many nonadherent dressings are available over the counter. Allowing the wound to dry and form a scab will delay healing. A slightly moist environment is preferable to a dry one. Apply a nonadherent dressing to the wound, and place an absorbent gauze dressing over it. Hold

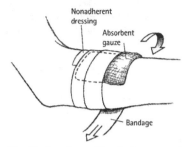

Fig. 61 *Dressing and bandaging a wound*

both dressings in place with a conforming roller bandage (**Fig. 61**).

:bulb: Weiss Advice

Making a Nonadherent Dressing

A nonadherent dressing can be made by spreading Polysporin or another antibiotic ointment over one side of a 10 x 10-cm (4 x 4-inch) gauze dressing. (Honey can be used in place of Polysporin. When applied topically, it can reduce infection and promote wound healing.)

A conforming roller bandage can be improvised from a shirt or other article of clothing by cutting a thin strip of material in a circular fashion.

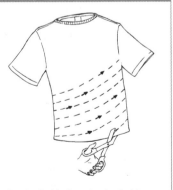

Cut the T-shirt in a circular fashion

Daily Wound Check

Check the wound daily for signs of infection. Even wounds closed under ideal circumstances have about a 5 percent chance of becoming infected, so check daily for the following signs of infection:

- Increasing pain, redness, or swelling
- Pus or greenish drainage from the wound
- Red streaks on the skin adjacent to the wound
- Fever

If signs of infection develop, remove the tape and open the wound to allow drainage. Pack the wound with moist gauze daily. Consult a physician as soon as possible, because antibiotics are usually given for wound infections.

Abrasions

An abrasion ("road rash") occurs when the outer layer of skin is scraped off. Abrasions are often embedded with dirt, gravel, and other debris that, if not removed, can result in scarring or infection.

An abrasion must be vigorously scrubbed with a surgical brush or cleansing pad until all foreign materials are removed. This can sometimes be more painful than the accident itself. It helps to first spread a topical anesthetic, such as 4% Xylocaine jelly, over the wound or to wipe the area with a cleansing pad containing lidocaine. Use clean tweezers to pick out any remaining embedded particles, then irrigate the abrasion with saline solution or water. A thin layer of aloe vera gel applied to the abrasion after cleaning will reduce inflammation and promote healing.

After cleansing, apply a nonadherent, protective dressing and secure it in place with a bandage. GlacierGel blister and burn dressings and

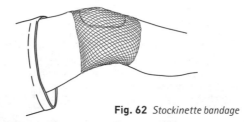

Fig. 62 *Stockinette bandage*

Spenco 2nd Skin both work well because they soothe and cool the wound while providing an ideal healing environment. GlacierGel dressings feature a 50% hydrogel dressing pad with an adhesive film layer attached for easy application. You can secure Spenco 2nd Skin with a stockinette or nonwoven adhesive knit bandage. Either dressing can be left in place for several days, as long as there is no sign of infection. A stockinette bandage is ideal for holding a dressing in place over a joint because it is stretchy, stays in place, and is less likely to allow sweat to build up (**Fig. 62**).

Blister Prevention and Treatment
Prevention
Eliminate as many contributing factors as possible:
- Make sure that shoes fit properly. A shoe that is too tight causes pressure sores; one that is too loose leads to friction blisters.
- Break in new boots gradually before a trip.
- Wear a thin liner sock under a heavier one. Friction will occur between the socks, instead of between the boot and the foot.
- Avoid prolonged wetness (wetness breaks down the skin, predisposing it to blister). Dry feet regularly and use foot powder.
- Before hiking, apply moleskin or Molefoam to sensitive areas where blisters commonly occur.

Hot Spots
Hot spots are sore, red areas of irritation, which, if allowed to progress, develop into blisters. Do the following to prevent a hot spot from progressing to a blister:

:bulb: Weiss Advice
Moleskin Substitute

If moleskin or Molefoam is not available, place a piece of tape over the hot spot (duct tape works well). Molefoam can be improvised from a piece of padding from a backpack shoulder strap or hip belt, while a piece of material from the cuff of a sweatshirt or flannel shirt can be used as moleskin.

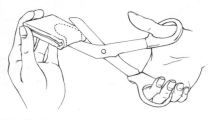

Fig. 63 *Cutting a doughnut hole in the middle of a piece of moleskin*

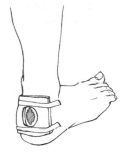

Fig. 64 *Covering a hot spot or blister with moleskin*

1. Take a rectangular piece of moleskin (soft cotton flannel with adhesive on the back) or Molefoam, which is thicker and somewhat more protective than moleskin, and cut an oval-shaped hole in the middle (like a doughnut) that is the size of the hot spot (**Fig. 63**).
2. Center this over the hot spot and secure it in place, making sure that the sticky surface is not on irritated skin. This will act as a buffer against further rubbing (**Fig. 64**).
3. Reinforce the moleskin with tape or a piece of nonwoven adhesive knit dressing.

☀ Weiss Advice

Gluing a Blister Back in Place

If you are far from help, must continue walking, and only have a tube of superglue or benzoin, consider this option: Drain the fluid from the blister with a pin or knife and inject a small amount of glue or benzoin into the space that you have evacuated. Press the loose skin overlying the blister back in place and cover the site with tape or a suitable dressing. The extreme pain this produces will only last a few minutes.

Treatment of Small, Intact Blisters

1. If the blister is small and still intact, do not puncture or drain it.
2. Place a piece of moleskin or Molefoam with a doughnut-style cutout slightly larger than the blister over the site. The covering should be thick enough to keep the shoe from rubbing against the blister. This may require several layers. Secure this with tape.

Treatment of Large or Ruptured Blisters

1. If the bubble is intact, puncture it with a clean needle or safety pin at its base, and massage out the fluid. The fluid contains inflammatory juices that can delay healing.
2. With scissors, trim away any loose skin from the bubble.
3. Clean the area with an antiseptic towelette or soap and water.
4. Apply antibiotic ointment or aloe vera gel, and cover with a non-adherent dressing or a gauze pad. Spenco 2nd Skin, GlacierGel blister and burn dressings, and Compeed hydrocolloid dressings are all excellent commercial blister dressings.
5. Place a piece of Molefoam, with a cutout slightly larger than the blister, around the site (**Fig. 64**). Secure everything with tape or a piece of nonwoven adhesive knit dressing. Change the dressing daily or every other day. First applying benzoin to the skin around the blister will help hold the Molefoam in place.
6. Inspect the wound daily for any sign of infection. (This includes redness around the wound, swelling, increased pain, or cloudy fluid collecting under the dressing.) If infection occurs, remove the dressing to allow drainage. Consult a physician as soon as possible.

BURNS

The severity of a burn injury is related to the size and depth of the burn and the part of the body that is burned. First-aid treatment and the necessity for evacuation are based on the overall burn size in proportion to the victim's total body surface area (TBSA).

The size of the burn injury can be estimated by the Rule of Nines or the Rule of Palms (**Fig. 65**).

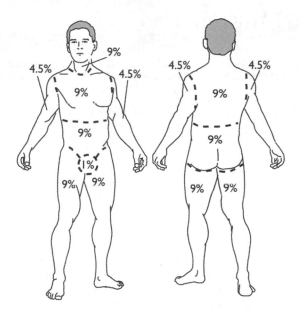

Fig. 65 *Rule of Nines body divisions*

Rule of Nines (Adults)

1. Each upper extremity = 9 percent of TBSA
2. Each lower extremity = 18 percent of TBSA
3. Front and back of trunk = 18 percent of TBSA (each)
4. Head and neck = 9 percent TBSA
5. Groin = 1 percent

Rule of Palms

An individual's palm covers an area roughly equivalent to 1 percent of his or her body surface area. Use the size of the victim's palm as a measure to estimate the percentage of body area burned.

⌖ When to Worry

Severe burns can lead to shock. With any of the following burns, evacuate the victim to medical care immediately:

- Second-degree burns greater than 20 percent total body surface area (TBSA)
- Third-degree burns greater than 10 percent TBSA
- Burns involving the hands, face, feet, or genitals
- Burns complicated by smoke inhalation
- Electrical burns
- Burns in infants and the elderly

People with facial burns, singed nasal hairs, coughs producing black spit, hoarseness, or wheezing should be evacuated immediately. They are in danger of developing an obstructed airway from severe swelling in the throat and windpipe.

General Treatment

1. Apply cool water to the area. Do not overcool the victim and produce hypothermia. (Use ice only on very small burns.)
2. Assess the airway, then do primary and secondary surveys.
3. Remove all burned clothing from the victim.
4. Remove any jewelry from burned hands or feet.
5. For chemical burns, flush the site with large amounts of water for at least 15 minutes.
6. A victim with a burn greater than 20 percent TBSA can lose a great deal of fluids from burned tissues and go into shock. If the victim is not vomiting and has a normal level of consciousness, encourage consumption of fluids.
7. Burns less than 5 percent TBSA (excluding second-degree burns of the face, hands, feet, genitals, or those that completely encircle an extremity) can be treated in the wilderness if adequate first-aid supplies are available and wound care is performed diligently.

First-Degree Burns (Superficial Burns)

Signs and Symptoms

Only the outermost layer of skin is involved in a first-degree burn. There is redness of the skin and pain, but no blisters are present. Sunburn is an example, as are most spilled-coffee burns.

Treatment

1. Cool the burn with wet compresses (do not use ice directly).
2. Apply aloe vera gel topically to the burn.
3. Anti-inflammatory drugs ibuprofen (Motrin) 600 mg three times a day with meals for 3 days) will provide pain relief and speed healing.
4. First-degree burns rarely require evacuation.

Second-Degree Burns (Partial-Thickness Burns)

Signs and Symptoms

A deeper burn resulting in both redness and blistering is considered a second-degree burn. Blisters may not occur for several hours following injury. The burned area is quite painful and sensitive to touch.

Treatment

1. Irrigate the burn gently with cool water to remove all loose dirt and skin.
2. Peel off or trim with scissors any loose skin.
3. Drain large—greater than 2.5-cm (1-inch)—thin, fluid-filled blisters and trim away the dead skin. Leave small, thick blisters intact.
4. Apply aloe vera gel or antibacterial ointment to the burn.
5. Cover the burn with a nonadherent dressing. Change the dressing at least once a day.

☀ Weiss Advice

Covering Burns with Honey

A gauze pad covered with honey is an effective covering for burns. It reduces infection and promotes healing of the wound.

Third-Degree Burns (Full-Thickness Burns)

Signs and Symptoms

Third-degree burns involve all layers of the skin, including nerves, blood vessels, and even muscle. Although these are the most serious burns, they are not painful, because the nerve endings have been destroyed. The skin next to a third-degree burn may have suffered only a second-degree burn and still be painful. The appearance of a third-degree burn is usually dry, leathery, firm, and charred when compared with normal skin, and it is insensitive to light touch or pinprick. Third-degree burns require skin grafting.

Treatment

1. Same as for second-degree burns.
2. Watch for shock.
3. Immediately evacuate the victim to a burn center.

MEDICAL EMERGENCIES: RESPIRATORY INFECTIONS

Tonsillitis ("Strep Throat")

Signs and Symptoms

Signs and symptoms that suggest bacteria (rather than a virus) as the cause of a sore throat include high fevers (over 39°C [102°F]), exudate or pus in the back of the throat, ("Hot Potato") a muffled voice, and enlarged lymph nodes in the neck.

Treatment

Bacterial sore throats are treated with antibiotics, such as penicillin or erythromycin.

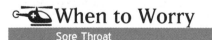 **When to Worry**

Sore Throat

If the victim cannot swallow his saliva or open his mouth fully, evacuate him immediately to a medical facility for treatment. Administer antibiotics, if available, en route (see Appendix D).

Sinus Infection (Sinusitis)

Infection of the sinuses may accompany a cold or hay fever.

Signs and Symptoms

The most prominent symptom is a frontal headache or feeling of heaviness above the eyes or adjacent to the nose. Drainage into the nose or back of the throat, nasal congestion, low-grade fever, and tenderness with pressing over the infected sinus are clues to a sinus infection. Pain may be felt in the upper jaw or teeth.

Treatment

Antibiotics (amoxicillin, Zithromax, Septra, doxycycline), decongestants, and antihistamines are recommended. The victim should seek medical care as soon as possible.

Bronchitis

Bronchitis is an infection of the air passages leading from the windpipe to the lungs. It is often caused by the same viruses that are responsible for colds.

Signs and Symptoms

The major symptom is a cough that may be dry or productive of yellow or greenish phlegm. Pain in the upper chest, which worsens with coughing or deep breathing, is sometimes present. Victims with bronchitis usually are not short of breath and do not have a rapid respiratory rate.

⌖ When to Worry

Cough

If shortness of breath, fever above 38°C (101°F), wheezing, severe pain in the chest, or a cough producing blood-specked or greenish phlegm is present, consult a physician as soon as possible.

Treatment
1. Cough expectorants that help bring up phlegm may be helpful. Cough suppressants such as codeine, which impair the body's normal process for expelling phlegm, should be reserved for nighttime use to allow for better sleep.
2. Drinking plenty of fluids will help thin the mucus and make it easier to expel.
3. Most cases of bronchitis are caused by viruses, which do not respond to treatment with antibiotics.

Pneumonia
Pneumonia is an infection of the lungs usually caused by either a bacteria or virus.

Signs and Symptoms
Symptoms include a cough that usually produces green or yellowish phlegm, fever, shaking chills, and weakness. Stabbing chest pain, often made worse with each breath, shortness of breath, and rapid breathing may also occur.

Treatment
Antibiotics (amoxicillin, erythromycin, Zithromax, Septra, Keflex, Cipro, or Levaquin) and professional medical care are needed. Zithromax is considered the antibiotic of choice.

SEIZURES
Seizures (or convulsions) can result from drugs, head injury, heat illness, low blood sugar, epilepsy, or other causes and, in children, fever.

Signs and Symptoms
Normally, a grand mal (full body) seizure lasts 2 to 3 minutes, during which the victim is unresponsive. When the seizure ends, the victim will be sleepy and confused and should be assisted to professional medical attention as soon as possible.

Treatment

1. Do not try to restrain convulsive movements.
2. Move harmful objects out of the way.
3. Make sure the airway is clear and the victim is breathing. If the victim is not breathing, start mouth-to-mouth rescue breathing.
4. If vomiting occurs, roll the victim onto his side to protect the airway.
5. Do not put anything in the victim's mouth.

INSULIN SHOCK AND DIABETIC KETOACIDOSIS

A diabetic who becomes confused, weak, or unconscious for no apparent reason may be suffering from insulin shock (low blood sugar) or diabetic ketoacidosis (high blood sugar).

Insulin Shock (Low Blood Sugar)

If a diabetic takes too much insulin or fails to eat enough food to match his insulin level or level of exercise, a rapid drop in blood sugar can occur.

Signs and Symptoms

Symptoms may come on very rapidly and include an altered level of consciousness, ranging from slurred speech, bizarre behavior, and loss of coordination to seizures and unconsciousness.

Treatment

If the victim is still conscious, give him something containing sugar to drink or eat as rapidly as possible, such as fruit juice, candy, or a nondiet soft drink. If the victim is unconscious, place sugar granules, cake icing, or glutose paste (should be in your first-aid kit if you or one of your companions is a known diabetic) under the tongue, where it will be absorbed rapidly.

Diabetic Ketoacidosis (High Blood Sugar)

Diabetic ketoacidosis (formerly called diabetic coma) comes on gradually and is the result of insufficient insulin. This eventually leads to a very high sugar level in the victim's blood.

Signs and Symptoms
Early symptoms include frequent urination and thirst. Later, the victim will become dehydrated, confused, or comatose and will develop nausea, vomiting, abdominal pain, and a rapid breathing rate with a fruity breath odor.

Treatment
The victim needs immediate evacuation to a medical facility. If vomiting is not present and the victim is awake and alert, administer small, frequent sips of water. If you are unsure whether the victim is suffering from insulin shock (low blood sugar) or ketoacidosis (high blood sugar), it is always safer to assume it is low blood sugar and to administer sugar.

HEART ATTACK
A heart attack occurs when the blood supply to the heart muscle is reduced or completely blocked due to an obstruction in one of the arteries supplying blood to the heart. If blood flow is not restored within 1 to 6 hours, part of the heart muscle will die.

Signs and Symptoms
The primary symptom of a heart attack is chest pain. The pain is usually a pressure, crushing, tightness, or squeezing sensation located in the center of the chest, and it may radiate up into the neck and jaw or shoulders or down the arms. Sometimes the victim experiences a burning sensation in the lower chest near the solar plexus or a feeling of indigestion. Cold sweats, nausea, vomiting, anxiety, shortness of breath, and weakness are often present.

Treatment
1. Have the victim chew or swallow one adult aspirin tablet (325 mg). Aspirin may help to partially open the blocked artery.
2. If the victim has nitroglycerin tablets, let him take them as prescribed.

3. If available, administer oxygen and pain medication to the victim.
4. Keep the victim in a comfortable position.
5. Arrange immediate evacuation to a medical facility with the patient doing as little as possible.

STROKE

A stroke is a life-threatening event in which an artery to the brain bursts or becomes clogged by a blood clot, cutting off the supply of oxygen to a part of the brain. A stroke can affect the senses, speech, behavior, thought patterns, and memory. It may also result in paralysis, coma, and death.

Signs and Symptoms
Any or all of the following may occur:

- Sudden weakness or numbness of the face, arm, and leg, usually on one side of the body (One side of the victim's mouth may appear to droop.)
- Loss of speech, slurred speech, or trouble talking or understanding speech
- Loss of vision in only one eye
- Sudden dizziness or loss of coordination
- Sudden onset of a severe headache

Treatment
Immediately transport the victim to a medical facility. Continually reassess the victim's airway and level of consciousness, as the condition can dramatically worsen during transport.

ABDOMINAL PAIN (BELLYACHES)

Abdominal pain can be due to many causes, including constipation, gas, infection, inflammation, internal bleeding, ulcers, and obstruction or aneurysms of major blood vessels. Abdominal pain can sometimes also be caused by pneumonia, a heart attack, kidney stones (see When to Worry, page 70), or pelvic problems.

⌁☤ When to Worry

Abdominal Pain

Seek medical help for any abdominal pain that lasts longer than 4 to 6 hours or is accompanied by frequent or projectile vomiting (vomit that seems to come out under pressure) or fever. Some common causes of abdominal pain that require urgent medical evaluation are appendicitis, ulcer, bowel obstruction, urinary tract and pelvic infections, and any pain during pregnancy.

Appendicitis

The appendix is located in the lower right side of the abdomen **(Fig. 66)**. Appendicitis occurs when the appendix becomes inflamed and swollen and fills with pus. Appendicitis can occur in persons of any age, but it is most common in young adults.

Signs and Symptoms

The victim usually has a vague feeling of discomfort that often begins in the center of the upper abdomen and within a matter of hours moves to the lower right side. Pain is persistent and steady but may be worsened by movement, sneezing, or coughing. There is usually loss of appetite, nausea, fever, and occasionally vomiting. Pressing on the stomach in the right lower quadrant increases the pain.

Treatment

Transport the victim to a hospital as soon as possible. Do not give the victim anything to eat. If evacuation will take longer than 24 hours and the victim is not vomiting, administer small sips of water at regular intervals (every 15 minutes). If available, administer a broad-spectrum antibiotic.

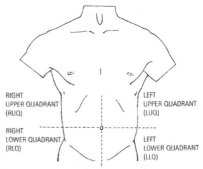

RIGHT UPPER QUADRANT (RUQ)

LEFT UPPER QUADRANT (LUQ)

RIGHT LOWER QUADRANT (RLQ)

LEFT LOWER QUADRANT (LLQ)

Fig. 66   *The four quadrants of the abdomen*

Ulcer

An ulcer is an erosion or crater that develops in the lining of the stomach or small intestine.

Signs and Symptoms

An ulcer usually produces persistent burning pain in the center of the upper abdomen, just below the solar plexus. The pain is occasionally relieved by eating and is often associated with nausea and belching. Dark black stools may indicate that the ulcer is bleeding. Sometimes an ulcer can be painless.

Treatment

1. Administer acid-reducing or acid-buffering medication, such as Maalox, Mylanta, Tagamet, Pepcid, or Zantac.
2. Avoid taking aspirin or anti-inflammatory drugs such as ibuprofen (Motrin).
3. Avoid alcohol, spicy foods, and tobacco.
4. Obtain medical evaluation as soon as possible.

☀ Weiss Advice

Ulcer Pain or Heartburn

When antacids are unavailable to treat ulcer pain or heartburn (acid indigestion), a glass of cold water alone will sometimes provide relief. A teaspoon or two of mentholated toothpaste, washed down, also may provide some relief. Avoid toothpaste brands that contain baking soda or hydrogen peroxide.

Bowel Obstruction

Bowel obstruction is a blockage of the intestines and occurs most commonly in individuals who have had previous abdominal surgery. It can also develop from infection or other causes.

Signs and Symptoms

Symptoms include nausea, vomiting, and cramping abdominal pain. The victim's breath may have a fecal odor, and the abdomen may look and feel distended.

Treatment

Evacuate the victim to a hospital. Do not give the victim anything to eat or drink.

Gallstones (Gallbladder Disease)

The gallbladder is connected to the underside of the liver in the upper right part of the abdomen (RUQ), just below the ribs. Stones can form in the gallbladder and produce an obstruction.

Signs and Symptoms

Pain and tenderness are present in the upper right side of the abdomen. Pushing under the rib cage on the right side of the abdomen while the victim takes a deep breath will increase the pain. The pain may radiate to the shoulder or back. Nausea and vomiting usually occur.

Treatment

Although the condition is not immediately life-threatening, it is best to evacuate the victim to a medical facility as soon as possible. Administer pain medication to the victim and broad-spectrum antibiotics if available. Do not give the victim anything to eat. If evacuation will take longer than 24 hours and the victim is not vomiting, administer small sips of water at regular intervals (every 15 minutes).

URINARY TRACT INFECTIONS

Bladder Infection

If you have to pull off the trail frequently to urinate and urinating is painful, then you most likely have a bladder infection. While a bladder infection is not usually a serious disease, it is very uncomfortable and, if untreated, can spread to the kidneys and produce a potentially dangerous kidney infection.

Women are much more likely to develop a urinary tract infection than men, because the tube that drains the bladder in women (urethra) is much shorter. The short female urethra allows infection-causing bacteria a shorter, easier trip to the bladder, where they can multiply and produce an infection.

Prevention
- Drink plenty of fluids to maintain a clear-looking urine.
- Don't postpone urinating when you feel the urge to go.
- Urinate immediately after sexual intercourse. This helps flush out any bacteria that may have accidentally been pushed into the urethra.
- *Women:* Wipe from front to back to avoid contaminating the urethral entrance with bacteria from the bowels.
- In hot or humid conditions, wear loose-fitting pants and wipe the perineal area frequently with moist towelettes.
- Drink cranberry juice to possibly prevent bladder infections. (Cranberry juice appears to inhibit the adherence of certain bacteria to bladder cells. Unfortunately, other fruit juices have not been found to share this medicinal quality.)

Signs and Symptoms
- Burning pain upon urination
- Urgent need to urinate frequently
- Cloudy, bloody, or bad-smelling urine
- Dull pain in lower abdomen

Treatment
Most bladder infections can be treated with a 3-day course of antibiotics such as Septra, Bactrim or Cipro. Another prescription drug, phenazopyridine hydrochloride (Pyridium), will help relieve pain and bladder spasms; it also turns urine and other body fluids reddish-orange, so don't wear contacts or expensive underclothes while taking it. Drink lots of fluids, especially cranberry juice if available.

Kidney Infection (Pyelonephritis)
Signs and Symptoms
Symptoms of a kidney infection may include those for bladder infection with the addition of back pain in the flanks, fever, chills, nausea, or vomiting.

Treatment
1. Initially treat the same as for bladder infections.
2. Evacuate the victim for medical care as soon as possible.

GYNECOLOGICAL EMERGENCIES
Vaginal Bleeding
Female travelers may experience a change in menstrual cycle due to stress. It is important to differentiate irregular vaginal bleeding or cessation of vaginal bleeding from pregnancy. If pregnancy is a possibility, seek medical help.

Any abnormal bleeding or abdominal pain accompanied by vaginal bleeding that is not associated with a normal menstrual period should be evaluated by a physician immediately. An ectopic, or tubal, pregnancy should be suspected if a menstrual period has been missed and vaginal bleeding and pelvic cramps develop. The condition can rapidly become life-threatening if not treated.

⚕🚁 When to Worry

Vaginal Bleeding

In a woman who is of childbearing age, any lower abdominal pain that is accompanied by vaginal bleeding and is not typical of a normal menstrual period should be evaluated for a possible ectopic pregnancy (abnormal pregnancy in a Fallopian tube). If a urine pregnancy test is negative, ectopic pregnancy is very unlikely. An ectopic pregnancy can be life-threatening if not emergently treated.

Gynecological Infections
Pelvic pain associated with fever, chills, nausea, vomiting, and weakness may indicate a pelvic infection. A yellow-green discharge may also be present. If immediate medical care is not available, start antibiotics right away (tetracycline 500 mg four times a day or doxycycline 100 mg twice a day, and metronidazole [Flagyl] 250 mg three times a day).

If a vaginal discharge is white and creamy (like cottage cheese) and is associated with vaginal or vulvar itching, and burning or pain on urination, the cause is usually vaginitis or a yeast infection. This can be treated with fluconazole (Diflucan) 150 mg taken orally, miconazole (Monistat), or clotrimazole (Gyne-Lotrimin) vaginal tablets (for 7 days) or cream (for 14 days). If none of these drugs is available, a vinegar douche can be helpful, as may airing the vaginal area and switching to cotton underwear or none at all. If the discharge is frothy, white-gray, and accompanied by abdominal pain and fever, the cause is often trichomoniasis. Treat with metronidazole (Flagyl) 250 mg three times a day for 5 to 7 days.

VOMITING

Treatment

Drink small but frequent amounts of a clear liquid, such as soup, 7UP, or half-strength Gatorade. To prevent the stomach from becoming distended and causing more vomiting, avoid drinking too much too soon. Avoid solid food until the vomiting has stopped.

When to Worry

Vomiting

Obtain professional medical care immediately if vomiting is associated with any of the following:
- Head or abdominal trauma
- Severe lethargy or confusion
- Severe abdominal pain or distention
- Blood in the vomit, or blood that looks like coffee grounds
- Fever higher than 38ºC (101ºF)
- Vomiting alone that continues for longer than 24 hours

DIARRHEA

Diarrhea is an increase in the frequency and looseness of stools. Causes of diarrhea include viruses, bacteria, parasites such as Giardia or Cryptosporidium, food allergies, inflammatory bowel disease, and anxiety.

Signs and Symptoms

A major concern with diarrhea is the amount of fluid loss or dehydration that results. The degree of dehydration can be estimated from certain signs and symptoms:

- **Mild dehydration** (3 to 5 percent weight loss): thirst; tacky mucous membranes (lips, mouth); normal pulse; dark urine
- **Moderate dehydration** (5 to 10 percent weight loss): thirst; dry

mucous membranes; sunken eyes; small volume of dark urine; rapid and weak pulse

- **Severe dehydration** (greater than 10 percent weight loss): drowsiness or lethargy; very dry mucous membranes; sunken eyes; no urine; no tears; shock (rapid pulse or one that is thready or difficult to feel)

⛑ When to Worry

Diarrhea

Obtain medical assistance if diarrhea is accompanied by any of the following:
- Blood or mucus in the stool
- A fever greater than 38°C (101°F)
- Severe abdominal pain or distention
- Moderate to severe dehydration
- Diarrhea lasting longer than 3 days

Treatment

1. Replace fluids and electrolytes. Oral rehydration with water and oral rehydration salts (ORS) is the most important treatment for diarrhea illnesses in the backcountry. The fluids and electrolytes lost from diarrhea can be potentially fatal in children and devastating in adults. The body has the ability to absorb the water and electrolytes given orally, even during a severe bout of diarrhea. Diarrhea fluid contains sodium chloride (salt), potassium, and bicarbonate, so plain water is an inadequate replacement. Many sport drinks sold commercially are not ideal for replacement of diarrhea losses: the high concentration of sugar may increase fluid loss, and the electrolyte contents may not be optimal. Gatorade can be used, but it should be diluted to half-strength with water.

2. The World Health Organization recommends Reduced Osmolarity ORS that contain the following combination of electrolytes added to 1 L (1 quart) of water: sodium chloride 2.6 g, potassium

chloride 1.5 g, glucose (anhydrous) 13.5 g, and trisodium citrate dihydrate 2.9 g.

3. Reduced Osmolarity ORS packets can be purchased commercially from Adventure Medical Kits, 800-324-3517, or improvised (see Weiss Advice, page 132).

4. Mildly or moderately dehydrated adults should drink 4–6 L (1–1.5 gallons) of ORS in the first 4 to 6 hours. Children can be given 240 mL (1 cup) of ORS every hour. Severe dehydration usually requires evacuation to a medical facility and intravenous fluids.

5. Rice, bananas, and potatoes are good supplements to oral rehydration solutions. Fats, dairy products, caffeine, and alcohol should be avoided. Full-strength juices should be avoided as a rehydration solution, since they usually contain three to five times the recommended concentration of sugar and can worsen the diarrhea.

6. *Antimotility drugs.* If the victim does not have bloody diarrhea or a fever greater than 38°C (101°F), loperamide (Imodium) can be taken orally to reduce cramping and diarrhea. The dose for adults is 4 mg initially, followed by 2 mg after each loose bowel movement, up to a maximum of 14 mg per day. Imodium is preferred over Lomotil, because it has fewer potential side effects. Imodium should not be given to children. Pepto-Bismol and Kaopectate are other commonly used antimotility drugs and may be helpful.

7. *Antibiotics.* Antibiotics are recommended if the diarrhea is accompanied by fever (38°C [101°F] or greater), if pus or blood is in the stool, if the victim has signs and symptoms of giardiasis (see "Giardiasis [Giardia]," page 132), or if the victim is traveling in a developing or underdeveloped country (see "Traveler's Diarrhea," page 133).

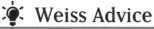

Weiss Advice

Rehydration Solutions

Try one of the following rehydration methods:

Rehydration Solution #1
    Add 6 g (1 teaspoon) table salt, 12 g (4 teaspoons) cream of tartar (potassium bitartrate), 2 g ($^1/_2$ teaspoon) baking soda, and 50 g (4 tablespoons) sugar to 1 L (1 quart) of drinking water.

Rehydration Solution #2
    Alternate drinking two separate solutions, prepared in the following manner:
- 250 mL (8 ounces) fruit juice, 2.5 mL ($^1/_2$ teaspoon) of honey or corn syrup, and a pinch of salt
- 250 mL (8 ounces) water and 1 g ($^1/_4$ teaspoon) baking soda

---

Giardiasis (Giardia)
Giardia is a hardy parasite that can thrive even in very cold water. Just one glass of contaminated water in the backcountry is enough to produce illness. Symptoms of giardiasis are usually delayed for 7 to 10 days after drinking contaminated water and may last 2 months or longer if the infection is not treated.

Signs and Symptoms
- Onset is usually gradual, with two to five loose or mushy stools per day.
- Stools are foul-smelling and contain mucus.
- The victim usually experiences a rumbling or gurgling feeling in the stomach and has foul-smelling gas, cramping abdominal pain, and nausea, and burps that taste like rotten eggs.
- General malaise and weight loss can occur.

Treatment
    Nitazoxanide (Alinia), a prescription medication, is now approved by the FDA for the treatment of giardiasis and has a better cure rate than metronidazole (Flagyl). The adult dose is 500 mg twice a day for 3 days.

The dose for children is 100 mg twice a day for 3 days. The adult dose of metronidazole is 250 mg three times a day for 7 days. In Asia and South America, tinidazole (Tiniba) is often used and can be taken as a single 2 g dose to cure the infection.

Cryptosporidiosis (Crypto)

Cryptosporidium (crypto) is a microscopic parasite similar to Giardia that lives in the feces of infected humans and animals. It is found in nearly all surface waters that have been tested nationwide. In 1995, more than 45 million Americans drank water from sources that contained Crypto. In Milwaukee in 1993, Crypto produced the largest outbreak of waterborne diarrhea in U.S. history.

Cryptosporidium is a resilient parasite. It is not killed by chlorine or iodine at concentrations normally used to disinfect drinking water and can slip through many water filters. The parasite is between 2 and 5 microns in size. Thus, filters must be able to remove particles smaller than 2 microns to be effective in eliminating Crypto from the water supply. Fortunately, the bug is vulnerable to heat and can be killed simply by bringing water to a full boil.

Signs and Symptoms

In most healthy people, Cryptosporidium causes abdominal cramps, low-grade fever, nausea, vomiting, and diarrhea, which can result in dehydration. Symptoms usually begin 2 to 7 days after drinking contaminated water and can last for up to 2 to 3 weeks before resolving on its own. For people with AIDS, on chemotherapy, or with a weakened immune system, Crypto may last for months and can be fatal.

Treatment

Nitazoxanide (Alinia) a prescription medication, is now approved by the FDA for the treatment of Cryptosporidiosis. The adult dose is 500 mg twice a day for 3 days. Loperamide (Imodium) may help decrease fluid loss and intestinal cramping.

Traveler's Diarrhea

Traveler's diarrhea refers to diarrhea that occurs in the context of foreign travel, usually in a developing country.

Prevention

Traveler's diarrhea is usually caused by bacteria and afflicts almost half of all visitors to underdeveloped countries. It is acquired through ingestion of contaminated food or water. Watching what you eat and drink may help but does not guarantee that you will not get sick. Travelers should avoid drinking untreated tap water as well as drinks with ice cubes. Bottled and carbonated drinks are generally safe. Custards, salads, salsas, reheated food, milk, and unpeeled fruits and vegetables should be avoided. Disinfected tap water should be used for brushing teeth.

Antibiotics are not recommended for prevention of traveler's diarrhea but are reserved for treatment if sickness occurs. Bismuth subsalicylate (Pepto-Bismol) is effective in preventing diarrhea in about 60 percent of travelers but must be taken in large quantities. 60 mL (4 tablespoons) four times a day, or 2 tablets four times a day, are needed. Unfortunately, this dosage contains a large amount of aspirin and can give some people stomach problems.

Signs and Symptoms

Symptoms usually begin abruptly 2 to 3 days after arrival. The diarrhea can be watery or soft, often with cramps, nausea, vomiting, malaise, and fever.

Treatment

1. See "Treatment" of diarrhea, page 130.
2. Antibiotics are effective for treating most cases of traveler's diarrhea. The best antibiotics are ciprofloxacin (Cipro) 500 mg twice a day for 2 to 3 days or azithromycin (Zithromax) 250 mg once a day for 2 to 3 days. Ciprofloxacin is not approved for use in children and may cause joint pain. A single dose of ciprofloxacin 750 mg or azithromycin 1000 mg is also effective. It is well worth a visit to a physician to obtain a prescription before a trip. Parts of Southeast Asia, such as Thailand, have bacteria that have become resistant to ciprofloxacin, and therefore azithromycin is recommended in these areas.

CONSTIPATION

Due to disruption of normal habits, constipation (difficult bowel movements with hard stools) is a common problem when traveling in the wilderness. Constipation is easier to prevent than to treat. Drinking fluids to stay well hydrated and adjusting the diet to include abundant fruits, vegetables, and whole grains are helpful preventive actions. If one becomes constipated, a stool softener can be used (mineral oil, Metamucil), with or without a gentle laxative such as prune juice or milk of magnesia. When no stool has been passed for 5 to 10 days due to constipation, the stool may have to be removed from the rectum using a gloved finger or enema. This should be done carefully to prevent injury to the anus and walls of the rectum.

HEMORRHOIDS

Hemorrhoids are enlarged veins found both outside and inside the anal opening. The best way to prevent hemorrhoids is to prevent constipation.

Signs and Symptoms

Hemorrhoids can cause minor itching, severe pain, and bleeding.

Treatment

Hemorrhoids can be treated topically with over-the-counter preparations such as Anusol or Preparation H. Any ointment with hydrocortisone will also be effective. Tucks hemorrhoidal pads with witch hazel are excellent for hemorrhoids (and also help to soothe poison ivy/oak rashes).

ALLERGIC EMERGENCIES

Allergic reactions can occur as a result of insect stings, food allergies, medications, exposure to animals, severe asthma, and other unknown reasons. Allergic reactions to insect stings are usually in response to the sting of a bee, wasp, hornet, or yellow jacket, or the sting of a fire ant. The most severe form of allergic reaction is anaphylactic shock, which can be life-threatening within minutes after contact with the substance to which the individual is allergic.

Severe Allergic Emergencies: Anaphylactic Shock

In anaphylactic shock, the victim may develop hives (red, raised skin welts), wheezing, chest tightness, shortness of breath, and a drop in blood pressure leading to dizziness, light-headedness, and fainting. The soft tissues of the throat, larynx, or trachea may swell, making it difficult or impossible for the person to swallow or breathe.

Treatment

The treatment for anaphylactic shock is epinephrine (adrenaline), and it must be given in the field. People allergic to bee stings or who have other serious allergies should carry injectable epinephrine with them at all times.

Obtaining epinephrine requires a prescription from your doctor. Epinephrine is available in the EpiPen and EpiPen Jr Auto-Injectors (0.3 and 0.15 mg epinephrine). These allow for self-administration of the medicine without a needle and syringe. Each device contains 2 mL of epinephrine 1:1000 USP in a disposable push-button, spring-activated cartridge with a concealed needle. The EpiPen will deliver a single dose of 0.3 mg epinephrine intramuscularly. The EpiPen Jr is used for children who weigh less than 30 kg (66 pounds); it delivers half the dose (0.15 mg epinephrine) of the adult injection. Instructions for use accompany the kits.

After administering epinephrine, give the victim oral diphenhydramine (Benadryl) 25 to 50 mg. Diphenhydramine is an antihistamine and may lessen the allergic reaction.

After treatment, transport the victim to a medical facility immediately, as an anaphylactic reaction can recur once the epinephrine wears off.

Mild Allergic Reactions

Not all allergic reactions are life-threatening. Often one may only develop hives (red, raised skin welts) and itching without wheezing or other breathing problems.

Treatment

Mild allergic reactions may be managed with an antihistamine such as diphenhydramine (Benadryl). The adult dose is 25 to 50 mg every 4 to 6 hours. The major side effect of this medication is drowsiness.

ASTHMA

Asthma, a respiratory disease involving the bronchial tubes in the lungs, can be life-threatening, especially in children. Many factors can predispose a susceptible individual to an attack, including pollen, animal hair, certain foods, upper respiratory infections, emotional stress, exercise, or exposure to cold air.

Signs and Symptoms

During an acute attack, the muscles around the small breathing tubes in the lungs tighten or constrict, causing wheezing, coughing, and the sensation of not being able to get enough air. Other symptoms of a severe attack include bluish tinge to the lips and fingers, rapid heartbeat, gasping for air, and confusion.

Treatment

Breathing medications that contain bronchodilators (e.g., albuterol) are most helpful during an attack. If the attack is severe, epinephrine from an EpiPen may be administered (as described on the previous page). Other useful medications include diphenhydramine (Benadryl) 50 mg and corticosteroids (prednisone 2 mg/kg). Evacuate the victim to a medical facility as soon as possible.

BITES AND STINGS

Venom from insects can produce severe allergic reactions and lead to life-threatening anaphylactic shock (see "Severe Allergic Emergencies," page 136). More commonly, insect bites and stings are painful and produce local reactions (redness, swelling) at the site.

General Treatment

1. Ice or cold packs will help alleviate local pain and swelling.
2. Sting relief swabs may help relieve pain when applied topically.
3. Oral antihistamines, such as diphenhydramine 25 to 50 mg (Benadryl) every 4 hours, are helpful in relieving the itching, rash, and swelling associated with many insect bites and stings.
4. The principles of wound care (see "Wounds: Cuts and Abrasions," page 102) apply to bites and stings as well. Any bite or sting can

become infected and should be examined at regular intervals for progressive redness, swelling, pain, or pus drainage.

5. Infectious diseases can be spread by insect bites and stings, especially in tropical and developing countries. Wearing protective clothing and applying insect repellents containing DEET are important preventive measures.

Bee Stings

Honeybees leave a stinger and venom sac in the victim after a sting. Hornets, yellow jackets, bumblebees, and wasps do not leave a stinger and may puncture a victim repeatedly.

Signs and Symptoms

Pain is immediate and may be accompanied by swelling, redness, and warmth at the site.

Treatment

1. If anaphylactic shock occurs, it must be treated immediately with epinephrine and antihistamines (see "Severe Allergic Emergencies," page 136).

2. After a honeybee sting, remove the stinger and venom sac as quickly as possible. Even with the rest of the bee gone, the venom sac can still continue to pump venom into your skin. *Do not hesitate or fumble for a pocketknife or credit card to scrape the stinger out of the skin.* It is better to grab the stinger and yank it out quickly than worry about pinching or squeezing more venom from the sac.

3. Apply ice or cold water to the sting site.

4. Anesthetic sprays, swabs, and creams may help relieve pain.

5. For adults, administer 25 to 50 mg diphenhydramine (Benadryl) for progressive itching, swelling, or redness.

🔆 Weiss Advice

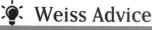

Taking the Sting Out of Bee and Wasp Venom

For bee venom (which is acid), apply a paste of baking soda and water. For wasp venom (which is alkaline), apply vinegar, lemon juice, or another acidic substance. Meat tenderizer applied locally to the sting site also may be effective in denaturing the venom and relieving pain and inflammation.

Black Widow Spider (Latrodectus mactans) Bites

Black widow spiders are black with a red hourglass mark on the underside of the abdomen and are about 16 mm (⅝ inch) long (**Fig. 67**). They like to hang out in woodpiles, stone walls, and outhouses. They generally are nocturnal.

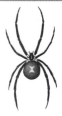

Fig. 67
Black widow spider

Signs and Symptoms

The bite of a black widow spider feels like a sharp pinprick but sometimes may go unnoticed. Within an hour, the victim may develop a tingling and numbing sensation in the palms of the hands and bottoms of the feet, along with muscle cramps, particularly in the abdomen (stomach) and back. In severe cases, the stomach muscles may become rigid and board-like. Sweating and vomiting are common, and the victim may complain of headache and weakness. High blood pressure and seizures can occur.

Treatment

Most people will recover in 8 to 12 hours without treatment. Small children and elderly victims, however, may have severe reactions, occasionally leading to death.

1. Apply ice packs to the bite to relieve pain.
2. Transport the victim to a medical facility as soon as possible.
3. Administer muscle relaxers such as diazepam (Valium), methocarbomal (Robaxin), or cyclobenzaprine (Flexeril) to help relieve muscle spasms.
4. A specific antidote is available for those suffering severe symptoms.

Brown Recluse Spider (Loxosceles reclusa) Bites
In the United States, the brown recluse spider
is found most commonly in the South and the
southern Midwest. The spider is brownish, with
a body length of 10 mm (just under 1/2 inch). A
characteristic dark, violin-shaped marking is
found on the top of the upper section of the body
(**Fig. 68**).

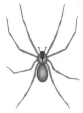

Signs and Symptoms

Fig. 68
Brown recluse spider

The bite sensation is initially mild, producing
the same degree of pain as an ant sting. The stinging subsides over 6 to 8 hours and is replaced by
aching and itching at the bite site. Within 1 to 5 hours, a painful red blister
appears, surrounded by a bull's-eye of whitish-blue discoloration. Over the
next 10 to 14 days the blister ruptures and a gradually enlarging ulcerated
crater develops, with further destruction of tissue. Fever, chills, weakness,
nausea, and vomiting may develop within 24 to 48 hours of the bite.

Treatment
1. Apply ice or cold compresses to the wound for pain relief.
2. If the blister has ruptured, apply a topical antibiotic ointment
   to the wound and cover with a nonadherent sterile dressing and
   bandage.
3. Get the victim to medical care as soon as possible. An antivenin is
   now available which, when used early, can prevent loss of tissue
   and scarring.

Tarantula Bites
Tarantulas are large, slow spiders.

Signs and Symptoms
A painful bite from a tarantula can sometimes become infected.

Treatment
1. Apply ice for pain relief.
2. Elevate and immobilize the bitten extremity to reduce pain.

3. Apply an antibiotic ointment to the site.
4. Take Motrin or Tylenol for pain, and antihistamines for itching.

Scorpion Stings

Scorpions, which are arthropods, are nocturnal and hide during the day under bark, in rocky crevices, or in the sand. Stings can be avoided by shaking out your shoes and clothes in the morning before dressing, not walking barefoot after dark, and by looking before picking up rocks or wood under which scorpions hide during the day.

Signs and Symptoms

Most North American scorpion stings produce only localized pain and swelling. The venom is injected by the stinger in the scorpion's tail. The pain of a nonlethal species is similar to that of a wasp or hornet, and the treatment is similar. Severe allergic reactions to scorpion stings are rare.

The potentially lethal scorpion found in the United States is *Centruroides sculpturatus,* also known as the bark scorpion, from its habit of hiding beneath loose and fallen pieces of tree bark. It is found in the desert areas of the southwestern United States (Arizona, New Mexico, California, and Texas) and northern Mexico. It is usually small (2 to 4 cm [1–2 inches] in length), straw-yellow in color, with long slender pincers, as opposed to bulky and lobsterlike. The venom contains neurotoxins that can be lethal but usually only in infants or small children.

The bark scorpion's sting causes immediate pain, which is worsened by tapping lightly over the bite site. Other symptoms include restlessness, muscle twitching that can sometimes look like a seizure, blurred vision, roving eye movements, trouble swallowing, drooling, slurred speech, numbness and tingling around the mouth, feet, and hands, and difficulty breathing.

Treatment

1. Place a piece of ice over the sting area to reduce pain.
2. Obtain professional medical care as soon as possible; an antivenin is available in the areas where lethal scorpions live.

Fire Ant (Solenopsis invicta) Bites
Fire ants are found in the southeastern states, Texas, and parts of California. They range in color from dull yellow to red or black. The ants are tenacious, and swarm and sting their victim repeatedly.

Signs and Symptoms
Initially, a cluster of small, painful, and itchy blisters develops. The blisters usually evolve into small pustules within 24 hours. The skin over the pustules, will slough away in 2 to 3 days, after which the sores heal. Some victims develop a severe reaction characterized by large, red, swollen welts that are very itchy. About 1 percent of stings are followed by severe allergic reactions.

Treatment
1. Apply ice or cold packs to the area.
2. Administer ibuprofin (Motrin) or acetaminaphen (Tylenol) with codeine for pain.
3. Treat the rash and itching with antihistamines such as Benadryl 25 to 50 mg every 4 to 6 hours. Topical steroid creams such as hydrocortisone or triamcinolone may also help to reduce the itching. In severe cases, a prescription for an oral steroid (prednisone) can be obtained from a physician, which will dramatically reduce itching.

Puss Caterpillar Stings (Megalopyge opercularis)
The puss caterpillar, or woolly slug, found in the southern United States has venomous bristles that inflict a painful sting.

Signs and Symptoms
Contact with a puss caterpillar causes instant pain, followed by redness and swelling at the site. Symptoms usually subside within 24 hours. In rare cases, nausea, headache, fever, vomiting, and shock may occur.

Treatment
1. Pat the skin with a piece of adhesive tape to remove any remaining bristles.
2. Apply hydrocortisone cream to the site to reduce itching, or take an oral antihistamine such as diphenhydramine (Benadryl).

Ticks

Ticks are brushed onto people who pass close-by. Once a tick lands on a person, it clings to hair or clothing and waits for several hours until the individual is at rest. Then it moves to an exposed area, often around the tops of the socks or at the neckline, attaches itself, and begins feeding.

Ticks secrete saliva and disease-producing organisms into the victim while feeding. About a hundred tick species transmit infections to humans. The most infamous are the tiny deer tick (*Ixodes scapularis*) and the blacklegged tick (*Ixodes pacificus*), which spread Lyme disease; the lone star tick (*Amblyomma americanum*), which transmits ehrlichiosis, Southern tick-associated rash illness (STARI), and tularemia; and the dog tick (*Dormacentor variabilis*), which transmits Rocky Mountain spotted fever, and tularemia.

Prevention

- Spray tents, sleeping bags, and clothing with permethrin, an insecticide that kills ticks before they have a chance to embed in your skin. Permethrin remains effective on your clothes for up to 2 weeks, and through several washings. It should not be used directly on the skin.
- Apply an insect repellent to your skin.
- Check yourself and your companions for ticks ("tick patrol") at least every 4 hours when in tick country.
- Wear long pants that are tucked into socks.
- Wear clothing that is light in color, making it easier to spot ticks.

Signs and Symptoms

An anesthetic agent in the tick's saliva usually makes the bite painless. Ticks feed from 2 hours to several days before dropping off.

Tick bites can occasionally produce a local reaction, a painful red and swollen wound at the puncture site, which can take a week or two to heal. The site can also become infected, requiring topical and oral antibiotics. If parts of the tick are left embedded in the skin, a painful nodule develops that then must be removed by surgical excision.

Some ticks carry a neurotoxin in their saliva, and on rare occasions a bite can lead to a temporary, or sometimes fatal, paralysis. Paralysis usually occurs only after prolonged attachment (more than 5 days) and begins in the legs and spreads to the arms and trunk and head. Removal of the tick stops the paralysis, and the victim recovers completely within several hours.

How to Remove an Embedded Tick

The tick should be grasped as close to the skin or surface as possible with tweezers, taking care not to crush, squeeze, or puncture the body (**Fig. 69**). Apply steady, straight upward traction to remove the tick. It may take a couple of minutes before the tick lets go. Avoid twisting, as the body can break off and leave the head still embedded in the skin. Tradi-

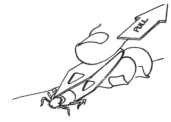

Fig. 69   *Removing a tick*

tional folk methods for removing ticks, such as applying fingernail polish, petroleum jelly, rubbing alcohol, or a hot match, increase the chance that the tick will salivate or regurgitate into the wound, thus spreading infection. After removal, clean the bite site with an antiseptic towelette.

Lyme Disease

Lyme disease is an infection caused by a spirochete, a type of bacteria that invades the body during the bite of an infected tick. Lyme disease is now the most common tick-transmitted infection, with an estimated 5000 to 15,000 new cases in the United States each year. The majority of people with Lyme disease do not recall the precipitating tick bite.

Lyme disease is most common in the Northeast (New York, Connecticut, Pennsylvania, New Jersey, and Rhode Island), in the upper Midwest (especially Michigan, Wisconsin, and Minnesota), and on the Pacific coast in California and Oregon. In areas of the Northeast, 90 percent of the deer ticks are infected with Lyme disease. In the West, only 1 to 2 percent of the ticks are infected.

Signs and Symptoms

Ranging from 3 days to a month (average of 7 days) after the tick bite, 70 percent of infected individuals develop an expanding, circular red rash. As the rash expands, it partially clears in the center, while the outer borders remain bright red, giving the appearance of a "bull's-eye." The rash can reach a diameter of 15 cm (6 inches) and may appear anywhere on the skin, unrelated to the bite site, although the thigh, groin, and armpit are the most common locations. The rash is warm to the touch and usually described by the victim as itching or burning, but it is rarely painful. It fades after an average of 28 days without treatment; with antibiotics, the rash resolves after several days.

Flulike symptoms such as fever, fatigue, headache, and muscle and joint aches, may develop before or with the rash, and last for a few days. About 20 percent of untreated people develop severe complications within weeks or months after the bite, ranging from heart and neurologic problems to severe attacks of arthritis (pain in the joints).

Treatment

If you develop a red rash after a tick bite in the backcountry, it is best to abort the trip and seek medical attention. The rash will help the physician diagnose Lyme disease and lead to early treatment with antibiotics.

VENOMOUS SNAKEBITES

Two classes of poisonous snakes are resident in the United States:

- Pit vipers (rattlesnakes, cottonmouths [water moccasins], and copperheads) have a characteristic triangular head; a deep pit (heat receptor organ) between the eye and nostril; and a catlike, elliptical pupil.
- Elapids (coral snakes) are characterized by their color pattern with red, black, and yellow or white bands encircling the body. The fangs are short—these snakes bite by chewing rather than by striking.

All states except Maine, Hawaii, and Alaska have at least one species of venomous snake. The states with the highest incidence of snakebites are North Carolina, Arkansas, Texas, Mississippi, Louisiana, Arizona, and New Mexico. About 90 percent of snakebites occur between April and October, because snakes are more active in warm months of the year.

The chance of dying from a venomous snakebite in the wilderness is extremely remote—about 1 in 12 million.

Most snakes can strike from a distance equal to about one-half their body length and may bite and not inject venom (dry bite); others can strike from a distance equal to their body length. No poisoning occurs in 20 to 30 percent of rattlesnake bites, and fewer than 40 percent of coral snake bites result in envenomation.

Pit Viper Envenomation

Signs and Symptoms

- One or more fang marks (rattlesnake bites may leave one, two, or even three fang marks)
- Local, burning pain immediately after the bite
- Swelling at the site of the bite, usually beginning within 5 to 20 minutes and spreading slowly over a period of 6 to 12 hours. (The faster the swelling progresses up the arm or leg, the worse the degree of envenomation.)
- Bruising (black-and-blue discoloration) and blister formation at the bite site
- Numbness and tingling of the lips and face, usually 10 to 60 minutes after the bite
- Twitching of the muscles around the eyes and mouth
- Rubbery or metallic taste in the mouth
- After 6 to 12 hours, possible bleeding from the gums and nose, denoting a serious envenomation
- Possible weakness, sweating, nausea, vomiting, and faintness

Treatment

The definitive treatment for snake venom poisoning is the administration of antivenin. The most important aspect of therapy is to get the victim to a medical facility as quickly as possible.

First Aid

1. Rinse the area around the bite site with water to remove any venom that might remain on the skin.
2. Clean the wound and cover with a sterile dressing.
3. Remove any rings or jewelry.

4. **Do not apply suction as first aid for snakebites. Suction has no benefit and may aggravate the injury.**

5. Apply a pressure immobilization bandage around the entire length of the bitten extremity as soon as possible. An elastic wrap bandage works best, but torn or cut strips of any flexible material, such as clothing or a towel, may be used. The wrap is started over the bite site and continued upward toward the torso in an even fashion, about as tight as one would wrap a sprained ankle. The wrap should not be uncomfortable, and it should be loose enough to allow a finger to be slipped under it. Do not take clothing off, as the movement of doing so might promote the movement of venom into the bloodstream. Extend the bandage as high as possible up the limb, but leave the tips of the fingers or toes unbandaged to allow the victim's circulation to be checked (**Fig. 70a–c**).

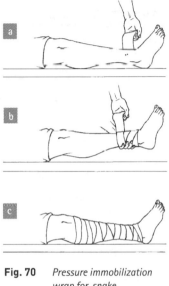

Fig. 70 *Pressure immobilization wrap for snake envenomation*

6. Immobilize the injured part as you would for a fracture, but splint it just below the level of the heart. If the bite is on a hand or arm, also apply a sling.

7. Transport the victim to the nearest hospital as soon as possible. If you pass by a telephone, stop and notify the hospital that you are bringing in a snakebite victim so staff can begin to locate and procure antivenin.

8. It is not necessary to kill the snake and transport it with the victim for identification. If the snake is killed, it should not be directly

handled but, rather, should be transported in a closed container. Decapitated snake heads can still produce envenomation.

Things Not to Do for a Snakebite

1. Do *not* make any incisions in the skin or apply suction with your mouth.
2. Do *not* apply ice or a tourniquet.
3. Do *not* shock the victim with a stun gun or electrical current.

Coral Snake Envenomation
Signs and Symptoms

- Burning pain at the site of the bite
- Numbness and/or weakness of a bitten arm or leg within 90 minutes
- Twitching, nervousness, drowsiness, increased salivation, and drooling within 1 to 3 hours
- Slurred speech, double vision, difficulty talking and swallowing, and difficulty breathing within 5 to 10 hours
- Possible paralysis

Symptoms may sometimes be delayed by up to 13 hours after the bite.

Treatment
The definitive treatment for snake venom poisoning is the administration of antivenin. The most important aspect of therapy is to get the victim to a medical facility as quickly as possible.

First Aid
First-aid treatment is the same as for a pit viper bite (see "Pit Viper Envenomation," page 146). Early use of the pressure immobilization technique is also highly recommended.

VENOMOUS LIZARDS
The Gila monster and Mexican beaded lizard are found only in the Great Sonoran Desert area in southern Arizona and northwestern Mexico. Both species possess venom glands and grooved teeth capable of

envenomating humans. Not all bites result in envenomation, since the lizard may only nip the victim or may not expel any venom during a bite.

A Gila monster may hang on tenaciously during a bite, and pliers or a sharp knife may be required to loosen the grip of its jaws.

Signs and Symptoms
- Pain and severe burning are felt at the wound site within 5 minutes and may radiate up the extremity. Intense pain may last from 3 to 5 hours and then subside after 8 hours.
- Swelling occurs at the wound site, usually within 15 minutes, and progresses slowly up the extremity. Blue discoloration may appear around the wound.

First Aid
1. Clean the wound thoroughly as you would for any laceration (see "Cleaning a Wound," page 104).
2. Inspect the wound and remove any shed or broken teeth.
3. Immobilize and elevate the extremity.
4. Obtain medical care as soon as possible.

OTHER ANIMAL BITES
Human or animal bites often become infected and can transmit diseases, such as rabies. Cat bites are especially prone to infection.

Treatment
1. Clean the wound vigorously (see "Cleaning a Wound," page 104).
2. The best antiseptic for bite wounds is benzalkonium chloride, because it helps to kill the rabies virus.
3. Never close an animal bite with sutures or tape. Pack the wound with saline-moistened gauze pads and cover with another dressing and bandage. Change the dressing daily.
4. Seek medical attention as soon as possible.

Rabies
Although rabies is uncommon (only 18 human deaths from rabies have occurred over the past 15 years in the U.S.), if not treated right away it will kill 100 percent of its victims. In the United States, raccoons, skunks,

and bats account for 96 percent of rabies cases, while foxes and coyotes make up most of the remaining cases. Any unprovoked attack by one of these animals should be considered an attack by a rabid animal.

Infection can occur even without a bite. The lick of an animal infected with rabies can transmit the disease if the saliva contacts an open wound or mucous membrane. There are even case reports of victims becoming infected with rabies after breathing the virus in bat-ridden caves. Squirrels, rats, mice, gerbils, chipmunks, and opossums have not been found to transmit rabies.

The rabies virus is transmitted to humans in the saliva of infected animals and attaches itself to nerves at the bite site. It then moves along the nerves to the brain. Because the virus causes no reaction until it reaches the brain, the infection goes unnoticed until it's too late. Once the virus has invaded the brain and symptoms develop, treatment is no longer effective, and death is inevitable.

The average time between the bite and the appearance of symptoms is 30 days. A bite on a leg allows more time for treatment than a bite on an arm because the virus has farther to travel to reach the brain. Bites about the face are particularly dangerous and must be treated immediately.

Signs and Symptoms

The initial symptoms of rabies infection are nonspecific and include malaise, fatigue, anxiety, agitation, irritability, insomnia, fever, head-ache, nausea, vomiting, and sore throat. After 2 to 10 more days, the victim may become aggressive, hyperactive, and irrational, and may develop seizures and hallucinations.

Treatment

1. Aggressively swab the wound thoroughly with benzalkonium chloride. If nothing else is available, scrub the wound vigorously with soap and water. Then irrigate the wound with lots of water.
2. If the biting animal can be safely captured, observe it for signs of rabies. If it's killed, the brain tissue can be tested for the virus.
3. The victim should seek the assistance of a physician as soon as possible. The doctor will determine the need for rabies vaccination (5 shots in the arm) and the administration of anti-rabies serum.

POISON IVY, POISON OAK, AND POISON SUMAC

Contact with poison ivy, poison oak, or poison sumac can cause an extremely itchy rash. The risk of developing a rash after exposure to these plants increases with each exposure. Your degree of sensitivity can change drastically from one exposure to the next. You may have a minor rash one year, then be incapacitated by a major breakout the next year. The offending resin is present in the plants year-round, even when they are only sticks or vines without leaves in winter.

In general, poison ivy grows east of the Rockies, poison oak grows west, and poison sumac grows best in the southeastern United States. These species do not grow in Alaska and Hawaii, nor do they survive well above 1200 m (4000 feet), in deserts, or in rain forests.

The leaflets on poison ivy and poison oak grow in clusters of three, leading to the saying "Leaflets three, let them be." Poison sumac leaflets grow in groups of seven to thirteen. The poison ivy vine can wind around a tree trunk or stretch across the ground. Poison oak is a low-growing shrub or woody vine. Poison sumac resembles a shrub or small tree.

IvyBlock, an over-the-counter cream, can provide some protection if placed on the skin at least 15 minutes before possible exposure to the plant. The cream is of no use if you already have the rash. Do not use this product on children younger than 6 years unless directed by a physician.

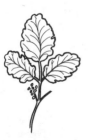

Poison oak

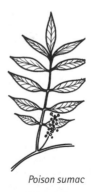

Poison ivy

Poison sumac

The resin binds to skin within 30 minutes. After that it cannot be washed off with soap and water. Some solvents such as Tecnu poison ivy cleanser or Zanfel may remove the oil from the skin even when used several hours after exposure. The sticky resin from any of these plants can stay active on clothing or shoes for many months, so handle contaminated clothing carefully and launder it immediately.

Signs and Symptoms

The rash may take a few hours to days to develop and starts as red, itchy bumps, followed by blisters that may become crusted. It can be streaky or patchy and "itches like crazy." It appears first where the concentration of resin was strongest and emerges over time on other areas of the body where it was less concentrated; this leads to the misconception that the oozing fluid from the skin spreads the rash. The rash cannot be spread by scratching after you have washed the original oil from the skin. Scratching is still discouraged because it can produce a secondary skin infection and actually increase itching.

Treatment

1. If left untreated, the rash will generally clear in about 2 weeks.
2. Topical over-the-counter steroid creams (such as 1% hydrocortisone cream) and calamine lotion may be useful for small patches of rash but are not effective if you have a severe case.
3. Cool, wet compresses made with Domeboro astringent solution may provide some relief from the itching.
4. Oral antihistamines such as diphenhydramine (Benadryl) 25 to 50 mg every 4 to 6 hours will help relieve some of the itching, but they also cause drowsiness.
5. For a widespread rash, or one involving the face or genitals, a physician can prescribe strong corticosteroid drugs such as prednisone, which can be taken orally or via injection. It takes about 12 hours for the drug to work, but once it does, the relief is dramatic. Side effects from a 2-week course of prednisone are generally mild and worth the benefit. The adult dose of prednisone for a severe case of poison oak or poison ivy is 100 mg for 2 days, 80 mg for 2 days, 60 mg for 2 days, 40 mg for 2 days, 20 mg for 2 days, 10 mg for 2 days, and 5 mg for 2 days.

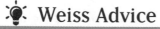 Weiss Advice

Removing Poison Oak or Poison Ivy from the Skin

Any solvent may help remove the oil of poison oak or poison ivy from the skin. Gasoline, paint thinner, and rubbing alcohol have all been reported to be effective. Note, however, that these products can themselves be irritating to the skin.

ALTITUDE ILLNESS (MOUNTAIN SICKNESS)

It is rare to experience altitude illness below 2400 m (6000 feet). Moderate altitude is between 2400 and 3600 m (8000 and 12,000 feet), high altitude is between 3600 and 5400 m (12,000 and 18,000 feet), and extreme altitude is over 5400 m (18,000 feet).

High-altitude illness is a direct result of the reduced barometric pressure and concentration of oxygen in the air at high elevations. Lower pressure makes the air less dense, so each inhalation contains fewer oxygen molecules so the body becomes deprived of oxygen.

Prevention

Graded ascent is the best and safest method of preventing altitude illness. Avoid abrupt ascent to sleeping altitudes greater than 3000 m (10,000 feet), and average no more than 300 m (1000 feet) of elevation gain per day above 3000 m (10,000 feet). Day trips to a higher altitude, with a return to lower altitude for sleep, will aid acclimatization. Eating foods that are high in carbohydrates and low in fat and staying well hydrated also help.

Acetazolamide (Diamox) is a prescription medication that may help prevent altitude illness when used in conjunction with graded ascent. Diamox works by increasing the respiratory rate, which is especially beneficial during sleep. It is also a diuretic (increases urination), so it has the potential to cause dehydration; thus, it is important to drink lots of fluids and be prepared for the inconvenience of getting up during the night to urinate. The dose for prevention is 125 mg the morning before arrival at altitude, again that evening, twice a day during ascent, and for at least 48 hours after reaching maximum altitude.

CAUTION: Before using Diamox, consult a physician. It can cause an allergic reaction in susceptible individuals and produce numbness and tingling in the hands and feet. Diamox will also ruin the taste of beer, cola, and other carbonated beverages.

Dexamethasone has been shown to prevent both *high-altitude cerebral edema* (HACE) and *high-altitude pulmonary edema* (HAPE) in a small study. The dose was 4 mg every 12 hours starting 2 days prior to exposure. Using dexamethasone, however, should generally be reserved for treatment of altitude illness and not for prevention.

Agents that block pulmonary hypertension may help to prevent HAPE. Nifedipine (Procardia), 20 mg sustained-release capsule every 24 hours, can prevent and ameliorate HAPE in susceptible individuals. Studies suggest that the inhaled beta-agonist salmeterol taken as 2 puffs every 8 to 12 hours via a metered-dose inhaler may prevent HAPE. Recent studies also suggest that sildenafil (Viagra) and tadalafil (Cialis) may also prevent HAPE by decreasing pulmonary artery pressure. Tadalafil, 10 mg twice a day, during ascent can prevent HAPE and is being studied for treatment.

Altitude illness can be divided into mild and severe forms.

The "Golden Rules" of Altitude Illness

1. Above 2400 m (8000 feet), headache, shortness of breath, nausea, or vomiting should be considered to be altitude illness until proven otherwise.
2. No one with mild symptoms of altitude illness should ascend any higher until symptoms have resolved.
3. Anyone with worsening symptoms or severe symptoms (HACE or HAPE) of altitude illness should descend immediately to a lower altitude.

Mild Altitude Illness: Acute Mountain Sickness

Signs and Symptoms

Acute mountain sickness (AMS) is common in travelers who ascend rapidly to altitudes above 2000 m (7000 feet). The typical sufferer experiences a headache, difficulty sleeping, loss of appetite, and nausea. Swelling of the face and hands may be an early sign. Children are generally more susceptible than adults.

Sleep is often fitful, with frequent awakenings and an irregular pattern of breathing, characterized by periods of rapid breathing alternating with periods of no breathing.

Treatment

1. When mild symptoms develop, one should not go any higher in altitude until the symptoms have completely resolved. Watch the victim closely for progression of illness to more severe forms. Usually, within 1 or 2 days, the victim will feel better and can then travel to higher altitudes with caution. Symptoms will improve more rapidly simply by going down a few thousand feet.
2. For headache, administer acetaminophen (Tylenol) 650 to 1000 mg or ibuprofen (Motrin) 400 to 600 mg.
3. Consider administering acetazolamide (Diamox) at a treatment dose of 250 mg twice a day.
4. Minimize exertion.
5. Avoid sleeping pills.

Severe Altitude Illness: High-Altitude Cerebral Edema (HACE)

Signs and Symptoms

A victim may experience one or more of the following:

- Severe headache unrelieved by Tylenol or Motrin
- Vomiting
- Loss of coordination
- Severe lassitude
- Confusion, inappropriate behavior, hallucinations, stupor, or coma
- Transient blindness, partial paralysis, or loss of sensation on one side of the body
- Seizures

Treatment

1. *Immediate descent* of at least 1000 m (3000 feet), or until the victim shows signs of considerable improvement, is the most important treatment. Do not wait to see if the victim gets worse or improves. Waiting could prove to be fatal.
2. Administer acetazolamide (Diamox) 250 mg twice a day.
3. Administer dexamethasone (Decadron) 8 mg followed by 4 mg every 6 hours if available.
4. Administer oxygen, if available.

5. When descent is not immediately possible, placing the victim in a portable hyperbaric chamber (Gamow bag) may be extremely beneficial. When zippered shut with the victim inside, this nylon bag is inflated with a foot pump, resulting in a significant decrease in altitude for the victim. Maintaining 2 psi inside the bag is equivalent to a descent of 1000 to 3000 m (3000 to 9900 feet), depending on the starting altitude. The bag takes approximately 2 minutes to inflate and is labor intensive; it requires 10 to 15 pumps per minute to maintain pressure and to flush out carbon dioxide. The total packed weight of a bag and pump is about 6.5 kg (14.3 pounds). The Gamow bag should not be used as a substitute for descent; it should be used when descent is not possible due to darkness, injury, or lack of people to carry a victim to a lower altitude.

When to Worry

Altitude Illness and Getting to Lower Altitudes

The single most useful sign for recognizing the progression of altitude illness from mild to severe is loss of coordination. The victim tends to stagger, has trouble with balance, and may be unable to walk a straight line heel to toe, as if drunk.

Progression of altitude illness symptoms, such as worsening headache or nausea—despite rest at the same altitude—or the development of loss of coordination, abnormal behavior, or confusion mandates immediate descent of about 1000 m (3000 feet), or until the victim shows signs of considerable improvement. Do not wait for morning to begin descent. An individual who might have been able to walk down under his own power with the aid of a headlamp can become a litter case in just 8 to 12 hours.

Never allow a victim to descend alone. Always have a healthy person accompany the individual.

Severe Altitude Illness: High-Altitude Pulmonary Edema (HAPE)
HAPE usually begins within the first 2 to 4 days of ascent to higher altitudes, most commonly on the second night.

Signs and Symptoms

A victim may experience one or more of the following:

- Marked breathlessness upon minor exertion
- A dry, hacking cough
- As fluid collects in the lungs, increasing shortness of breath, even while resting, and a cough that may produce frothy sputum
- Anxiety, restlessness, and a rapid, bounding pulse
- Cyanosis (a bluish color of the lips and nails, indicating poor oxygenation of the blood)

Treatment

1. *Most important:* Immediate descent of at least 1000 m (3000 feet), or until the victim shows signs of considerable improvement. Do not wait. Waiting could be fatal.
2. Administer oxygen, 4 to 6 liters per minute, if available.
3. The prescription drug nifedipine (Procardia) may be helpful for HAPE. The dose is 10 to 20 mg every 8 hours.
4. The use of the Gamow bag (described on the previous page) may be beneficial when the victim cannot be immediately evacuated to a lower altitude.

FROSTNIP, FROSTBITE, AND IMMERSION FOOT
Prevention

Frostbite occurs in cold and windy weather conditions. Even if the temperature outdoors is not very cold, high winds can reduce the effective temperature to a dangerously low level. The chilling effect of air at 20°F moving at 64 km/h (40 miles an hour) is the same as at -20°F on a still day.

On long trips it is important to drink often to prevent dehydration and to eat often to provide fuel so the body can generate heat. If the body is cold and dehydrated, it will shunt blood away from the skin, predisposing an individual to frostbite.

Other things that predispose one to frostbite and that should be avoided are smoking, tight restrictive clothing and shoes, and contact of bare flesh with cold metal. Individuals with diabetes, known sensitivity to cold, or poor circulation are more likely to suffer frostbite.

☀ Weiss Advice

Windmilling for Warmth

If you feel your fingers getting numb from the cold, swing your arms around in a circle like a windmill for a few minutes. Windmilling increases blood flow to the hands and fingers and may delay the onset of frostbite.

Frostnip

Frostnip (also called superficial frostbite) is an early cold injury to the skin and does not usually lead to permanent damage. It may progress to deeper frostbite if left untreated.

Signs and Symptoms

Frostnip is usually characterized by numbness of the involved area. Common locations are the fingers, toes, nose, and earlobes. The affected parts will initially appear red, then turn pale or whitish. Frostnipped parts are still soft and pliable to the touch.

Treatment

1. Rewarm frostnipped areas immediately to prevent the progression to frostbite. Self-treatment includes placing the fingers in one's own armpit or groin and leaving them there until they are warm and no longer numb. Bared feet may also be placed on the warm stomach of a companion.
2. Chemical heat packs are also beneficial. Take care not to burn the skin with them.

Frostbite

Frostbite is freezing of the skin and usually indicates that some degree of permanent damage has occurred.

Signs and Symptoms

Frostbite is recognized by skin that is white and waxy in appearance. The frostbitten part feels hard, like a piece of wood.

Treatment

The best treatment for frostbite is rapid rewarming in warm water as soon as the victim can be maintained in a warm environment. Rapid rewarming is preferable to slow rewarming because the damage to tissue occurs during the actual freezing and thawing phases. If possible, avoid rewarming the frostbitten area if there is a danger of refreezing. Walking on frozen feet to shelter is much less damaging than walking on feet that have been thawed. Allowing the feet to refreeze again after thawing is the worst possible scenario.

1. Rapidly rewarm frozen extremities in water at a temperature of 40–41°C (104–106°F). Circulate the water to keep the involved part in contact with the warmest water, and avoid rubbing or massaging the skin. Keep checking the water temperature, as it will cool quickly. Add more hot water as needed. Remove the extremity from the water before adding more hot water. Thawing in warm water usually requires 30 to 45 minutes of immersion and can be very painful. If pain medication is available, administer a dose to the victim before beginning. Thawing is complete when the paleness has turned to a pink or red color and the skin is soft.

2. After thawing, the involved part will be very sensitive to further injury and should be protected. Application of aloe vera gel to the skin has been shown to be beneficial in promoting healing of frostbitten skin.

3. When frostbite is rewarmed, fluid-filled blisters (blebs) may form. If this occurs, remove the loose skin overlying the blister and apply aloe vera or antiseptic ointment.

4. Place small sterile gauze pads between toes or fingers, cover the injury with a nonadherent sterile dressing, and loosely wrap the extremity with a bulky bandage.

5. Administer ibuprofen (Motrin) 600 to 800 mg every 12 hours to help relieve pain and possibly minimize tissue loss.

6. Elevate and splint the affected part.

The depth and degree of the frozen tissue cannot be readily determined by looking at the body part. Even terrible-looking limbs often recover if treated well, so reassure the victim and seek professional medical care as soon as possible.

Things *Not* to Do for Frostbite

- Do *not* rub the affected part with snow. In fact, do not massage, rub, or touch the frozen part at all.
- Be careful *not* to use water that is hotter than 41°C (106°F) because a burn injury may result.
- Do *not* use any type of tobacco. Nicotine markedly reduces blood flow to the fingers and toes.
- Do *not* thaw the frozen extremity in front of a fire or stove.
- Do *not* let the thawed extremity refreeze.
- When possible, do *not* walk on frostbitten feet or use frostbitten fingers, as that will cause further injury.

Immersion Foot (Trench Foot)

Trench foot occurs in response to exposure to nonfreezing cold and wet conditions over a number of days, leading to damage of blood vessels, nerves, skin, and sometimes muscle without complete freezing of tissues.

Signs and Symptoms

- Numbness and a pins-and-needles sensation may occur in the feet.
- During the first few hours to days, the feet become very red and swollen and then mottled with dark red to blue splotches.
- The feet can become extremely painful after rewarming and very sensitive to cold and touch.

Treatment

Keep the feet dry and warm and treat as you would for frostbite, with the exception that rapid rewarming (thawing) is not necessary.

HYPOTHERMIA

Hypothermia is an abnormally low body temperature due to exposure to a cold environment. Core (rectal) temperature down to 32°C (90°F) is considered mild to moderate hypothermia, while temperatures below this indicate profound or severe hypothermia. When the body's temperature falls below 28°C (83°F), the heart becomes irritable and is prone to lethal irregularities, such as ventricular fibrillation. Death from hypothermia is likely to occur at around 24–27°C (75 to 80°F). The lowest recorded core temperature in a surviving adult is 16°C (60.8°F); for a child, it is 14°C (57°F).

Although few people freeze to death in the backcountry, fatal accidents and injuries resulting from hypothermia-induced poor judgment and incoordination are all too common.

Hypothermia is often divided into mild and profound cases, based on a victim's temperature and behavior (see Table 2, page 163). The distinction is important, because the treatment and the worry factor are different. It can be hard to tell where one level starts and the other stops without a special low-reading thermometer. Certain signs and symptoms can often be used to gauge a victim's level of hypothermia.

How We Lose and Conserve Heat

Radiation: Direct loss of heat from a warm body to a cooler environment. The head and neck account for more than 50 percent of the body's heat loss. Protective clothing, including a hat and scarf or neck gaiter, will help prevent this heat loss.

Conduction: Heat loss through direct physical contact between the body and a cooler surface. Insulating someone from the ground will help prevent this type of heat loss.

Convection: Heat loss by air movement circulating around the body, with the amount of loss depending on the wind velocity (windchill factor). Windproof clothing and shelter will help reduce this type of heat loss. In a survival situation, wrapping a garbage bag around the victim or even using a pack as a bivy sack can help protect from wind chill.

Evaporation: Sweat or water evaporating or drying on your skin cools the body. This type of heat loss can be minimized by using a vapor barrier liner under clothing. Less recognized is the cooling effect of evaporation from breathing. This can be reduced by breathing through a scarf or face mask.

Mild Hypothermia
At 35°C (95°F), a victim is mildly hypothermic.

Signs and Symptoms
- The victim feels cold, and shivering reaches its maximum level.
- The victim maintains a normal level of consciousness, is alert, and has normal or only slightly impaired coordination.
- At 34°C (93°F), the victim develops apathy, amnesia, slurred speech, and poor judgment.

Treatment
1. Get the victim into shelter and insulate him from the cold.
2. Replace any wet clothing with dry, insulated garments.
3. Give the victim warm food and lots of sugar-containing fluids to drink. Elevating the core temperature of an average-size individual 1°F requires consuming about 60 kilocalories worth of a hot beverage. Because a quart of hot soup at 60°C (140°F) provides

---

Your Body's Thermostat Is in Your Skin!

Your perception of whether you are cold or warm depends more on your skin temperature than on your core temperature. Even when your core temperature is above normal, if your skin is cold you will feel cold and begin shivering (an involuntary condition in which your muscles twitch rapidly to generate additional body heat). Conversely, if your core temperature is low but your skin is warm, you feel warm, and you do not shiver, despite being hypothermic.

This underappreciated concept is important to understand if you spend time in the wilderness. If you warm a hypothermic individual's skin without providing any heat to the core (e.g., putting a chemical heat pad on the skin), you can extinguish the drive to shiver and cause the blood vessels on the skin to dilate, which will make a person more hypothermic.

It is known that profoundly hypothermic victims sometimes rip off their clothes prior to death. This phenomenon (paradoxical undressing) occurs because the constricted blood vessels near the body's surface suddenly dilate when the core temperature reaches a certain level and produce a sensation of warmth at the skin.

Table 2
Hypothermia Table

BODY TEMPERATURE-RELATED FINDINGS*	
Core Temperature	**Characteristics**
37.2°C (99°F)	Normal rectal temperature
37°C (98.6°F)	Normal oral temperature
35°C (95°F)	Maximum shivering
33.8°C (93°F)	Poor judgment; slower movements
33°C (91.5°F)	Clumsy movements; apathy
31°C (88°F)	Shivering stops; stupor; altered level of consciousness
28.3–30°C (83–86°F)	Heart is irritable and prone to arrhythmias
26.6°C (80°F)	Voluntary motion ceases; pupils not reactive to light
22.2–25°C (72–77°F)	Maximum risk of cardiac arrest
*General guidelines only; marked variations may occur	

about 30 kilocalories, a victim would have to consume 2 L (2 quarts) to raise core temperature 1 degree F. The sugar content of the fluid, however, will provide added fuel for the victim's furnace for generation of internal heat.

4. Heat loss may be slowed by wrapping the victim in plastic bags, tarps, or sleeping bags. Huddling together will reduce heat loss.
5. Resist the urge to use hot water bottles or heat packs; they can turn off the shivering mechanism and, by themselves, add very little heat to the core. Instead, bring water to a boil and have the victim inhale the steam, or build a fire.

Profound Hypothermia
At 32°C (90°F), a victim is profoundly hypothermic.

Signs and Symptoms

- The victim becomes weak and lethargic and has an altered mental state (disorientation, confusion, combative or irrational behavior, or coma).
- The victim is uncoordinated (unable to walk a straight line, heel to toe, without stumbling).
- At 31°C (88°F), the victim will stop shivering.
- At 30°C (86°F), the victim's heart pumps less than two-thirds the normal amount of blood. Pulse and respirations will be half of normal.
- At 28.3°C (83°F), the heart is very irritable and unstable and prone to developing irregularities, such as ventricular fibrillation. The victim is in danger of sudden cardiac arrest; rough handling of the victim increases the potential for this to happen.

Treatment

First-aid treatment is aimed at preventing further cooling and stabilizing the victim.

1. Handle the victim gently. Rough handling may cause the victim's heart to fail.
2. Place the victim in a sleeping bag, or place blankets or clothing underneath and on top of him. Any heat that you can provide will probably not rewarm the victim but will help prevent further cooling.
3. Do not allow a victim with a significantly altered mental state to eat or drink because of the potential for choking and vomiting.
4. Rewarming is best done in a hospital because of the potential complications associated with profound hypothermia. Professional assistance is usually needed to evacuate a profoundly hypothermic victim.

CAUTION: First-aid management of hypothermic victims should not be based solely on measurements of body temperature, because obtaining an accurate temperature in the field can be difficult. It is only one consideration, along with other observations and signs (such as an altered mental state) that are used in guiding decision making about appropriate treatment.

It may be difficult to distinguish between someone who is profoundly hypothermic and someone who is dead. The profoundly hypothermic person may have a pulse and respirations that are barely detectable. Because the heart rate may be very slow, double-check carefully, feeling for the carotid pulse for at least 1 full minute in a hypothermic victim. Place a cold glass surface next to the victim's mouth to see if it fogs up.

When to Perform CPR for Hypothermia

If the victim is breathing or has any pulse, no matter how slow, do not initiate CPR. If there is no sign of a pulse or breathing after 1 minute, what to do next depends on your situation.

- If you're alone or with only one other person, cover and place the victim in a protected shelter with insulation above and below. Stay with the other rescuer for safety, including going for help.
- If there are multiple rescuers, and it is safe to stay with the victim, begin CPR while at least two people go for help.

Never assume that a profoundly hypothermic victim is dead until the body has been warmed and there are still no signs of life. Rarely, a victim who is without detectable signs of life, and presumed to be dead, will recover when rewarmed.

HEAT ILLNESS

Heat emergencies encompass a spectrum of illnesses, ranging from such minor reactions as muscle cramps to heatstroke, which is a life-threatening emergency.

Some days it is better to stay in the shade or camp indoors next to an air conditioner. The potential for developing heat illness is greatest in an environment that is both hot and humid. When the outside temperature exceeds 35°C (95°F), evaporation of sweat from the body's surface is the only mechanism left to dissipate heat. If the humidity level then exceeds 80 percent, the ability to lose heat (from evaporation) declines dramatically, and the risk of developing heat illness soars. Sweat that merely drips from the skin and is not evaporated contributes to dehydration without providing any cooling benefit.

Prevention

Keep yourself hydrated. Dehydration is the most important contributing factor leading to heat illness. When you're overheated, the blood vessels near the skin dilate so that more blood can reach the surface and dissipate heat. If you're dehydrated, the blood vessels in the skin will constrict and you will not be able to cool off readily.

More important, dehydration limits the ability of the body to sweat and evaporate heat.

Unfortunately, the body's dehydration sensor is not very sensitive. It waits until we're already 2 to 5 percent dehydrated before sounding the thirst alarm and then shuts off prematurely, after we have replaced only two-thirds of the fluid defect. The best way to tell if you're hydrated is by urine color:

- Clear to pale-yellow urine indicates that you're drinking enough fluids.
- Dark, yellow-colored urine indicates dehydration. (Note: Some vitamins and medications can also turn urine a yellow/orange color.)

During exercise, you can easily sweat away 1–2 L (1–2 quarts) of water per hour. Trying to keep yourself hydrated requires a continual, conscious effort. Carry your water bottle where it is easily accessible and drink at least 0.5 L (1 pint) every 20 minutes during a hike. As a general rule of thumb in a hot environment, a person should drink 4 L (1 gallon) of water for every 20 miles walked at night and 8 L (2 gallons) for every 20 miles walked during the day.

The colder and tastier the beverage is, the more likely you will want to drink it. Wrap the container in an article of clothing to help keep it cool, and add a powdered sports drink mix after disinfecting the water. Your body can absorb a carbohydrate-containing beverage up to 30 percent faster than plain water. Diluted Gatorade (one-third to half strength) is ideal. Higher carbohydrate concentrations should be avoided, because they can produce stomach cramps and delay absorption.

Salt lost in sweating can usually be replaced by a normal diet or by adding a small amount of salt to your drinking water. The ideal concentration is a 0.1 percent salt solution, which can be prepared by crushing and then dissolving two 10-grain salt tablets or 1.5 g (¼ teaspoon) of table salt in 1 L (1 quart) of water. Do not eat salt tablets by themselves; they irritate the stomach, produce vomiting, and do not treat the dehydration that is also present.

- *Hike in the early morning and late afternoon* when the sun is low and the heat less intense.
- *Avoid certain medications and drugs:*
    1. Antihistamines found in many cold and allergy preparations decrease the rate of sweating.

2. Antihypertension drugs such as beta-blockers, ACE inhibitors, and diuretics can predispose you to heat illness.
3. Amphetamines, PCP, and cocaine can all cause heat illness by increasing metabolic heat production.

▦ *Allow yourself adequate time to acclimatize before exercising* for prolonged periods in the heat. It takes about 10 days to become acclimatized to a hot environment. During that time, you will need to do about 2 hours of exercise each day. With acclimatization, your body becomes more efficient at cooling itself and you are less likely to suffer heat illness.

▦ *Wear clothing that is lightweight and loose-fitting for ventilation, and light-colored to reflect heat.*

▦ *Get plenty of rest.* A U.S. Army study found a correlation between lack of sleep, fatigue, and heat illness.

Heat Exhaustion
Heat exhaustion is the most common form of heat illness.

Signs and Symptoms
▦ Malaise, headache, weakness, nausea, and loss of appetite
▦ Vomiting
▦ Dizziness when standing up from a sitting or lying position
▦ Dehydration
▦ Core temperature ranging from normal to moderately elevated (to 40°C [104°F])
▦ Sweating, normal mental state, continued coordination

Treatment
1. Stop all exertion and move the victim to a cool and shaded environment.
2. Remove restrictive clothing.
3. Administer oral rehydration solutions with plenty of water.
4. Place ice or cold packs alongside the neck and chest wall, under the armpits, and in the groin. Fanning while splashing the skin with tepid water, or soaking the victim in cool water, are other cooling methods.

WARNING: Do not place ice directly against the skin for prolonged periods.

Heatstroke

The difference between heatstroke and heat exhaustion is that victims with heatstroke have abnormal mental states and neurological functions. They can be confused or display erratic or bizarre behavior, be disoriented, or seem off-balance (the victim may appear intoxicated and be unable to walk a straight line). Seizures and coma are late manifestations. Sweating may still be present in heatstroke. Dry, hot skin is a very late finding and may not occur in some victims. Therefore, those who have a temperature above 40°C (105°F) and an altered mental state should be considered to have heatstroke whether or not they are still sweating.

Signs and Symptoms

- Elevated temperature (usually above 40°C [105–106°F])
- Altered mental state (confusion, disorientation, bizarre behavior, seizures, coma)
- Rapid heart rate
- Low blood pressure
- Rapid respiration
- Sweating present or absent

Treatment

1. Cool the victim as quickly as possible. Place ice or cold packs alongside the neck and chest wall, under the armpits, and in the groin, where large blood vessels come near the surface. Wet the victim's skin with tepid water, and fan the victim rapidly to facilitate evaporative cooling. Immerse the victim in cool water if available.
2. Do not give the victim anything to drink because of the risk of vomiting and aspiration.
3. Do not give acetaminophen or aspirin, as they are not helpful in heatstroke.
4. Treat for shock (see "Shock," page 32).
5. Evacuate the victim immediately to the closest medical facility.

Continue to cool along the way until the victim's temperature falls to 38°C (100–101°F).

6. Recheck the temperature at least every 30 minutes.

🔆 When to Worry

Heatstroke

Heat exhaustion that is not treated can progress to full-blown heat-stroke, which is a life-threatening medical emergency. Anyone suffering from heat illness who has an altered mental state (loss of coordination, bizarre behavior, confusion) should be treated for heatstroke with rapid cooling, and transported to a hospital.

Heat Edema

Swelling of the hands, feet, and ankles is common during the first few days in a hot environment. It is usually self-limited and does not require any treatment.

Prickly Heat

The rash of prickly heat is caused by plugged sweat glands in the skin.

Signs and Symptoms

An itchy, red, bumpy rash develops on areas of the skin kept wet from sweating.

Treatment

1. Cool and dry the involved skin and avoid conditions that may induce sweating for a while.
2. Antihistamines such as diphenhydramine (Benadryl) may relieve itching.

Heat Cramps

These painful muscle spasms or cramps usually occur in heavily exercised muscles.

Signs and Symptoms

Spasms often begin after exertion has ended and a person is resting.

Treatment
Prevention and treatment consist of drinking plenty of fluids containing small amounts of salt (see "Heat Illness," page 165). Salt tablets taken alone are not advised. Rest in a cool environment and apply gentle, steady pressure to the cramped muscle.

Heat Syncope
When a person stands for a long time without moving, blood pools in the legs instead of returning to the heart. Standing in a hot environment also causes blood vessels on the surface of the skin to dilate, taking more blood away from the heart, which means there is less blood traveling to the brain.

Signs and Symptoms
The combined effects of heat syncope can cause someone to faint from insufficient blood flow to the brain.

Treatment
Lying in a horizontal position with the legs elevated (Trendelenburg position) and cooling the skin will treat this condition.

DIVING MEDICINE
Near Drowning
Treatment
1. If a drowning victim is not breathing, mouth-to-mouth rescue breathing is the only first-aid treatment that matters (see "Rescue Breathing," page 25). Do not perform a Heimlich maneuver unless you are unable to breathe air into the victim because of an obstructed airway. A Heimlich maneuver will not drain water from the lungs and may produce vomiting and aspiration.
2. Expect the victim to vomit during rescue breathing. When he does, logroll him onto his side and sweep out the vomitus from his mouth. Then roll him back over and continue the resuscitation.
3. Note evidence of trauma and immobilize the spine if indicated by the mechanism of the event (see "C2: Cervical Spine Protection," page 21).
4. Check for a pulse and begin chest compressions if necessary.

5. Remove the victim's wet clothing and cover him with blankets or other dry, warm material to prevent hypothermia. Be sure to protect the victim from conductive heat loss by also placing material between him and the ground or other cold surface.

6. Take all victims of a near drowning to a hospital for evaluation, even if they appear fully recovered. Delayed worsening of lung functioning may occur.

Following drowning in cold water less than 10°C (50°F), several victims have been revived even after 20 minutes of submersion (and two have survived more than one hour). These remarkable saves are presumably due to the protective effects of profound hypothermia. If possible, perform CPR on cold-water drowning victims until they reach the hospital or until help arrives.

Air Embolism

An air embolism follows a rupture in the lungs between the air space and the blood vessels that carry blood back to the heart. When an air embolism occurs, bubbles of air are released into the arterial bloodstream. This can lead to a stroke, heart attack, headache, and/or confusion. An embolism usually occurs when a diver ascends too rapidly without adequately exhaling.

Signs and Symptoms

Symptoms and signs of an air embolism may include unconsciousness, confusion, seizures, or chest pain after surfacing. Any symptoms that appear in a previously normal diver more than 10 minutes after surfacing are probably not due to an air embolism.

Treatment

Anyone suspected of having an air embolism should be placed in a head-down position (with the body at a 15- to 30-degree tilt) on the left side. Assist with mouth-to-mouth breathing if necessary, and immediately transport the victim to a medical facility. The treatment for air embolism is recompression in a hyperbaric chamber. When available, oxygen can be administered at a rate of 10 L (10 quarts) per minute by face mask.

Decompression Sickness (Bends)

When a diver descends in the water, nitrogen present in the compressed air is absorbed by the body. If a diver ascends too rapidly, microscopic bubbles of nitrogen exit the bloodstream into the surrounding tissue, causing "the bends."

Signs and Symptoms

Symptoms can begin immediately after ascent or may develop over a period of hours. Symptoms include joint pain, numbness and tingling of the arms and legs, back pain, fatigue, weakness, inability to control the bladder or bowel, paralysis, headache, confusion, dizziness, nausea, vomiting, difficulty speaking, itching, skin mottling, shortness of breath, cough, and collapse.

Treatment

Treat anyone suspected of having the bends with immediate oxygen therapy (10 liters per minute by face mask). Transport the victim to the nearest medical facility. Professional treatment for the bends is recompression in a hyperbaric chamber. Divers should not fly for 12 hours after a no-decompression dive and for 24 hours following a decompression dive.

Nitrogen Narcosis

At depths greater than 27 m (90 feet), divers are at risk for this disorder, caused by the absorption of nitrogen into the bloodstream.

Signs and Symptoms

Symptoms include confusion, euphoria, bad judgment, and unconsciousness.

Treatment

Never dive alone. Assist a diving partner exhibiting any symptoms of nitrogen narcosis to the surface.

Ear Squeeze

If a diver cannot equalize the pressure on the eardrum by forcing air through the Eustachian tube and into the middle ear, the eardrum stretches inward and may rupture. A rupture allows water to enter the middle ear.

Signs and Symptoms
Ear squeeze results in pain, dizziness, nausea, vomiting, and disorientation.

Treatment
A diver with ear squeeze should remain calm and slowly ascend to the surface. The ear should be allowed to dry on its own. Insert nothing into the ear, as it may increase the damage to the eardrum. Obtain immediate medical assistance.

Sinus Squeeze
Sinus squeeze commonly occurs when a diver cannot equalize sinus pressure, due to nasal congestion during descent, and the sinuses contract. (A "reverse squeeze" occurs during ascent, when air expands in the sinus. This can be very painful but will resolve itself.)

Signs and Symptoms
- Pressure or pain in the forehead or around the teeth, cheeks, or eyes may occur.
- The nose may bleed.
- Pressure and pain increase with depth.

Treatment
1. If a sinus squeeze occurs, slowly ascend to the surface.
2. Apply warm compresses to the face.
3. Take nasal decongestants such as oxymetazoline (Afrin) and oral decongestants such as pseudoephedrine (Sudafed).
4. Oral antibiotics (ampicillin, erythromycin, or azithromycin [Zithromax]) are recommended if sinus pressure persists or if there is a discharge from the ear or nose.

HAZARDOUS MARINE LIFE

Many types of marine life can be hazardous to unwary victims. People spending time near the ocean should be aware of the potential dangers presented by the marine life residing there. One of the best ways to avoid problems associated with hazardous marine life is to become familiar with the creatures that cause problems and learn how to avoid them.

Sharks

Shark bites can cause severe damage or death, usually through blood loss and shock (see "Wounds: Cuts and Abrasions," page 102). Even small shark bites should be examined by a physician. Any animal bite presents high risk for infection and should not be sewn or taped tightly shut. Allow the wound to drain and begin antibiotic therapy (doxycycline [Vibramycin] or trimethoprim/sulfamethoxazole [Septra]).

Sharks also have very rough skin and can impart a nasty scrape. Treat the victim as you would for a second-degree burn (see "Second-Degree Burns," page 117).

Barracudas and Moray Eels

Treat both these types of bites as you would a shark bite.

Corals and Barnacles

To avoid infection from coral and barnacle cuts and scrapes, scrub the area vigorously with soap and water, then flush the wound with a large amount of water. Continue by flushing with a half-strength solution of hydrogen peroxide and water. Rinse the area again with clean water. Apply antibiotic ointment and cover the wound with a nonadherent dressing. Clean the wound twice daily. If the wound shows any sign of infection (increased redness, pus, swollen lymph glands, or red streaks near the wound), consult a physician. Antibiotic therapy includes trimethoprim/sulfamethoxazole (Septra), ciprofloxacin (Cipro), or tetracycline.

Sponges

Contact with sponges can lead to a rashlike reaction characterized by redness, itching, and swelling. Treat by soaking the affected area with vinegar (5% acetic acid) for 10 to 15 minutes. Dry the skin, and repeatedly apply and remove sticky adhesive tape to the area to remove any embedded sponge spicules. Repeat the vinegar soak for 5 minutes or apply rubbing alcohol for 1 minute. Apply hydrocortisone cream 1% two times a day until the irritation is resolved.

Jellyfish

Jellyfish inflict painful, occasionally life-threatening, stings. Stings occur when the skin comes into contact with jellyfish tentacles, which contain millions of venomous stinging cells. Broken-off pieces of jellyfish that wash up on the beach can remain toxic for months and should not be handled. The venom from the box jellyfish (from northern Australia) can kill in minutes by causing abnormal heart rhythms and cardiopulmonary collapse. The symptoms and treatment for jellyfish stings are to some degree similar to those for the Portuguese man-of-war (bluebottle), box jellyfish (sea wasp), Irukandji jellyfish, fire coral, stinging hydroid, sea nettle, and sea anemone.

Signs and Symptoms

Symptoms range from mild burning and redness to severe pain and blistering. Victims may also experience nausea, vomiting, shortness of breath, and low blood pressure.

Treatment

1. Immediately apply vinegar (5% acetic acid). If vinegar is not available, flush the area with sea water. Cold packs or ice may relieve pain following a man-of-war sting. Do not rinse with fresh water or apply ice directly to the skin.
2. Apply vinegar (5% acetic acid) or rubbing alcohol (40 to 70 percent) for 30 minutes or until the pain subsides. If these products are not available, use household ammonia (one-fourth strength). Urine and meat tenderizer have limited usefulness.
3. Remove any embedded particles using a Splinter Picker or tweezers. Be careful not to touch the fragments with your bare hands.
4. Apply shaving cream or a baking soda paste. Shave the area using a razor or other sharp-edged object.
5. Reapply the vinegar or alcohol soak for 15 minutes.

6. Apply a layer of hydrocortisone cream 1% two times a day.
7. Seek medical attention if a large area is affected, if the victim is very old or very young, or if you observe significant signs of illness (nausea, vomiting, weakness, shortness of breath, chest pain, etc.).
8. If the victim was stung on the mouth or has any respiratory tract involvement, do not give anything by mouth. Monitor the condition constantly to ensure an unobstructed airway, and transport the victim to definitive medical care.
9. If the sting is from the Australian box jellyfish, seek immediate assistance in addition to completing the above steps. An antivenin is available.

Sea Urchins

Sea urchin spines are venomous. The puncture wounds from these animals can cause difficulty in breathing, weakness, or collapse. To treat this injury, immerse the affected area in hot water to tolerance 43–45°C (110–113°F). Carefully remove only visible spines. Do not attempt to clean the wound thoroughly. Consult a physician. If the victim shows any signs of infection, administer trimethoprim/sulfamethoxazole (Septra), ciprofloxacin (Cipro), or tetracycline.

Sea Cucumbers

Treat any skin irritation resulting from contact with a sea cucumber the same as for a jellyfish sting. If the eyes are involved, flush with at least 1 L (1 quart) of water. Seek immediate medical attention.

Stingrays

Injury from a stingray includes both deep puncture wounds or lacerations and envenomation. Symptoms include pain, bleeding, weakness, vomiting, headache, fainting, shortness of breath, paralysis, collapse, and, on occasion, death. Rinse the wound with water (fresh or sea water). Immerse the area in hot water to tolerance 43–45°C (110–113°F) for 30 to 90 minutes. Scrub the wound well with soap and water. Do not attempt to close the wound: a serious infection could result. If a physician is more than 12 hours away, administer an antibiotic (trimethoprim/sulfamethoxazole (Septra), ciprofloxacin (Cipro), or tetracycline).

Catfish
Treat as you would a stingray wound. Hot water can provide significant pain relief.

Scorpionfish
Treat the same as a stingray wound. Seek immediate medical attention if the victim appears intoxicated (weak, vomiting, short of breath, or unconscious). In Australia, an antivenin is available.

Sea Snakes
Sea snakes bite with four fangs. The venom can cause paralysis, destruction of red blood cells, and generalized muscle damage. The site of the bite may not be very painful. If symptoms do not develop within 6 to 8 hours of a bite, venom is not present to any great degree in the wound. Symptoms include weakness, paralysis, lockjaw, drooping eyelids, vomiting, darkened urine, difficulty speaking, and difficulty breathing. Treat this emergency as you would a land snakebite (see "Venomous Snakebites," page 145).

Swimmer's Itch, Seaweed Dermatitis, and Seabather's Eruption
While these conditions are caused by different entities, the treatment is the same. Skin reactions, including red, itchy areas, often with blisters and/or weeping, develop after swimming. This can be treated by washing with soap and water, followed by a rinse of isopropyl (rubbing) alcohol 40 to 70 percent. Apply hydrocortisone cream 1% two times a day. If the reaction is severe or persists, see a doctor.

Fish Handlers' Disease
This infection usually starts in small nicks or cuts on fish handlers' hands. It is characterized by a skin rash erupting 2 to 7 days after exposure. Usually the skin surrounding the cut will appear red or violet colored and will be slightly warm and tender. Treatment includes antibiotic therapy (penicillin, cephalexin (Keflex), or erythromycin).

SEAFOOD POISONING
Scromboid Poisoning
Scromboid poisoning results from eating contaminated fish (usually tuna, mackerel, bonito, skipjack, mahimahi, anchovies, sardines, or Australian ocean salmon). The fish may or may not have a peppery or metallic taste.

Signs and Symptoms
Almost immediately after eating the fish, the victim will develop symptoms similar to an allergic reaction, including becoming flushed, itching, hives, abdominal pain, nausea, diarrhea, and a low-grade fever.

Treatment
Treat this reaction with diphenhydramine (Benadryl) every 6 to 8 hours until it resolves.

Paralytic Shellfish Poisoning
Paralytic shellfish poisoning is a serious illness caused by eating shellfish contaminated with algae that contains a toxin harmful to humans. All molluscan shellfish, including clams, mussels, oysters, and scallops, can contain paralytic shellfish poison.

Signs and Symptoms
Minutes after eating contaminated shellfish, the victim may experience tingling and numbness of the lips and mouth, light-headedness, and weakness. Symptoms also include drooling, difficulty swallowing and breathing, incoordination, headache, thirst, diarrhea, abdominal pain, blurred vision, sweating, and rapid heartbeat. Death can result in as little as 2 hours, as muscles used for breathing become paralyzed.

Treatment
Treatment for severe cases is supportive and may require the use of a mechanical respirator. Seek medical care as soon as possible.

FISHHOOK INJURIES

Fishhooks have a barb just behind the tip and are curved so that the more force applied to the hook, the deeper it penetrates. The barb prevents the hook from being backed out. The classic method of advancing the barb through the skin and cutting the hook so that the remaining shank can be backed out is effective, but there is an easier and less painful technique.

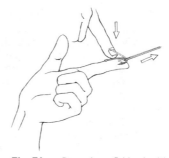

Fig. 71   *Removing a fishhook with the string technique.*

Removing a Fishhook

Pass a length of string, fishing line, suture material, or dental floss through and around the bend of the hook. Grasp the ends of the string and, while applying gentle downward pressure on the shank to disengage the barb, yank on the string (**Fig. 71**).

After removing the hook, clean the entry point with an antiseptic towelette or soap and water.

CAUTION: Fishhooks embedded in the eye should be left in place and secured with tape, the eye covered with a metal patch or cup, and the victim transported to an ophthalmologist for definitive care.

LIGHTNING INJURIES

In an average year, lightning kills more people in the United States than either tornadoes or hurricanes. Carrying or wearing metal objects, such as an ice axe, umbrella, backpack frame, or even a hairpin, increases the chances of being hit.

To calculate the approximate distance in miles from a flash of lightning, count in seconds from the time you see the flash to when you hear the thunder, then divide by five.

The Four Mechanisms of Lightning Injury

1. *Direct hit.* Lightning directly strikes a person in the open. It usually does not enter the body but instead is conducted over the
   skin surface "flashover", producing a variety of injuries. The
   greatest damage may occur to skin beneath metal objects worn
   by the victim, such as jewelry, belt buckles, or zippers, which tend
   to disrupt the flashover and allow current to penetrate. Current
   may also penetrate the body through the eyes, ears, and mouth,
   causing deeper injuries to those parts. The victim is exposed to a
   tremendous electromagnetic field, which can disrupt the work-
   ings of the brain, lungs, and heart and lead to cardiac and respiratory arrest. Finally, the instant vaporization of any moisture on
   the victim's skin can blast apart clothing and shoes.
2. *Splash.* A more common scenario is for the victim, to be struck by
   lightning "splash," which occurs when a bolt first hits an object,
   such as a tree or another person, and then "jumps" to the victim,
   who may have found shelter nearby. Splashes may also occur from
   one person to another when they are standing close together.
3. *Step voltage.* Lightning hits the ground or a nearby object, and the
   current spreads like a wave in a pond to the victims. Step voltage
   is often to blame when several people are hurt by a single lightning bolt.
4. *Blunt trauma.* The explosive force of the pressure waves created
   by lightning can cause blunt trauma, such as spleen or liver injuries and ruptured eardrums.

Types of Lightning Injuries

1. *Heart and lung.* Lightning can cause a cardiac arrest and paralyze
   the lungs. The heart will often restart on its own, but because the
   lungs are still not working, the heart will stop again from lack of
   oxygen.
2. *Neurological injuries.* The victim may be knocked unconscious
   and suffer temporary paralysis, especially in the legs. Seizures,
   confusion, blindness, deafness, and inability to remember what
   happened may result.
3. *Traumatic injuries.* Bruises, fractures, dislocations, spinal injury,

and chest and abdominal injuries from the shock wave may occur. Ruptured eardrums can result in hearing loss.

4. *Burns.* Superficial first- or second-degree burns are more common than severe burns after a lightning strike and form distinctive fern patterns on the skin.

Prevention

- When a thunderstorm threatens, seek shelter in a building or inside a vehicle (not a convertible).
- Occupants of tents should stay as far away as possible from the poles and all wet fabric, including clothing.
- Do not stand underneath a tall tree in an open area or on a hilltop.
- Get out and away from open water.
- Get away from tractors and other metal farm equipment.
- Get off bicycles and golf carts.
- Stay away from wire fences, clotheslines, metal pipes, and other metallic paths that could carry lightning to you from some distance.
- Avoid standing in small, isolated sheds or other small structures in open areas.
- In a forest, seek shelter in a low area under a thick growth of saplings or small trees. In an open area, go to a low place, such as a ravine or valley.
- If you are totally in the open, stay far away from single trees to avoid lightning splashes. Drop to your knees, bend forward, and put your hands on your knees. If available, place insulating material (e.g., sleeping pad, life jacket, rope) between you and the ground. Do not lie flat on the ground.

Treatment

Lightning strike victims are not "charged" and thus pose no hazard to rescuers.

1. The immediate treatment of lightning strike victims differs from other situations with multiple trauma victims. Rather than adhere to the standard rescue dogma of ignoring the victims who appear dead, and giving priority to those who are still alive,

after a lightning strike treat those victims first who appear dead, because they may ultimately recover if quickly given mouth-to-mouth rescue breathing and CPR. If you're successful in obtaining a pulse with CPR, continue rescue breathing until the victim begins to breathe spontaneously or you are no longer able to continue the resuscitation.

2. Stabilize and splint any fractures.
3. Initiate and maintain spinal precautions if indicated.

PREPARING FOR FOREIGN TRAVEL

Nearly one-half of travelers to developing countries become ill during their visit. Diseases such as polio, malaria, and typhoid fever that are uncommon in the United States are a threat to travelers who visit areas where poor sanitation and contaminated food and water exist. International travelers should contact their local health department, physician, or travel medicine clinic at least 6 weeks prior to departure to obtain current health information on countries they plan to visit and to begin receiving vaccinations. Beside vaccinations, travelers should undergo medical and dental exams prior to departure and should obtain prescription medications that may be needed during travel (see Appendix D). The Centers for Disease Control and Prevention (CDC) Travelers' Health website provides help in locating clinics for pretravel consultation. The site also provides links to state health departments and the Yellow Fever Vaccination Center Registry, which lists facilities approved to provide yellow fever vaccinations (wwwnc.cdc.gov/travel /page/find-clinic.htm).

The CDC provides travel health information to address the many different health risks a traveler may face with electronic access through its website (www.cdc.gov/travel). This site offers information to assist travelers in deciding the vaccines, medications, and other measures necessary to prevent illness and injury during international travel. *CDC Health Information for International Travel* (The Yellow Book) is the most trusted resource for travel health and is available in a searchable online version on the CDC Travelers' Health website (wwwnc.cdc.gov/travel).

The World Health Organization (WHO) also maintains recommendations regarding vaccine requirements for international travelers, with its annual publication of vaccination requirements and health advice in *International Travel and Health*, with electronic access through its website (www.who.int/ith).

Timing of Vaccines

Travelers should begin receiving vaccinations at least 6 weeks prior to departure. Travelers often request vaccinations at the last minute, leading to concerns about the appropriate timing and spacing of injections. In general, inactivated vaccines or toxoids, such as those for hepatitis B, cholera, typhoid, rabies, plague, influenza, tetanus, diphtheria, or inactivated polio, may be given simultaneously at separate sites.

Live vaccines, such as those for measles, mumps, rubella, and oral polio, can be administered simultaneously with an inactivated vaccine, except those for cholera and yellow fever. Immune globulin given for hepatitis A can be given simultaneously with inactivated vaccines and toxoids. Live vaccines should be given at least 2 weeks before immune globulin or 3 to 5 months afterward.

Required Vaccine

Yellow Fever (YF) is an acute viral hemorrhagic disease transmitted to humans by mosquitoes in tropical Africa and South America. YF transmission occurs in jungle and urban cycles in South America, with peak transmission during the months of January, February, and March.

Countries located in YF endemic areas—including certain countries in Africa (Burkina Faso, Cameroon, Congo, Côte D'Ivoire, Democratic Republic of Congo, Gabon, Ghana, Liberia, Mali, Mauritania, Niger, Rwanda, São Tomé, Togo) and one in South America (French Guiana)—require proof of YF vaccination from all arriving travelers.

The vaccine is a live attenuated virus. The immunization must be given no less than 10 days prior to the planned date of entry. Vaccine administration is documented and stamped on the appropriate page of the International Certificate of Vaccination. This proof of vaccination is sometimes required during crossing of international borders, particularly in Africa, or if flying from an infected country to a noninfected country, even if the stay in the endemic country was a brief transit stop.

YF vaccine is approved for use in all persons over 9 months of age who have no YF vaccine contraindication. The primary schedule for YF vaccine in adults is a single 0.5 mL injection given subcutaneously. The duration of immunity from one dose of the vaccine is estimated to last for 10 years or longer. A booster dose is recommended for persons with continued risk of exposure 10 years from the last dose.

YF vaccine can be administered concurrently or at any time before or after immune globulin products given for hepatitis A prophylaxis.

Recommended Vaccines

Diphtheria, Pertussis, Measles, Mumps, Rubella, Varicella, and Polio are childhood immunizations that all international travelers should keep up to date. Tetanus should be updated with a booster every 10 years. Travelers born after 1956 who have not received two doses of measles vaccine or do not have a well-documented history of having the illness as a child should receive a single injection of the measles vaccine. Travelers who have previously completed a primary polio series and have never had a booster should receive a booster dose of oral polio vaccine (OPV). Cases of measles and varicella have been reported as travel-acquired infections among international travelers, and these common childhood infectious diseases are known to cause more serious disease in infections acquired by adults.

Cholera Vaccine

The highest incidence of cholera cases in the world is being reported from Africa (predominantly from South Africa, Democratic Republic of Congo, Mozambique, and Malawi).

Cholera vaccine is not required for entry into any country under current WHO International Health Regulations. Cholera vaccine is not recommended for short-term tourists traveling to an endemic country. Immunization may be recommended for travelers who plan extensive travel or work in highly endemic/epidemic areas under unsanitary conditions and without access to Western-style medical care.

The newer cholera vaccines are the live attenuated oral vaccines and killed whole cell (KWC) oral vaccines. The live attenuated oral cholera CVD 103-HgR vaccine is extremely safe. The vaccine should not be given to immunosuppressed people or those with chronic liver disease. There are no data available on safety in pregnant women. The killed whole cell oral cholera vaccine also appears to be extremely safe; the only contraindication is intolerance to a previously administered dose.

The KWC vaccine is taken in 2 doses separated by 7 to 42 days. A booster is recommended every 2 years for repeated exposure.

Hepatitis A Vaccine

Hepatitis A is a viral infection transmitted by contaminated food or water or by direct person-to-person contact. Hepatitis A is one of the most common vaccine-preventable infections acquired during travel. The risk of hepatitis A infection is highest in developing countries with poor sanitation and food hygiene. Most travel-related cases (72 percent) have been associated with travel to Mexico and Central/South America.

Hepatitis A vaccine (Havrix) is recommended for travelers going to developing countries where sanitation may be poor. The vaccine is given as a single injection to adults and as 2 injections one month apart to children under 17 years of age. A booster injection 6 to 12 months later is also recommended. It takes at least 3 weeks to be protected after the initial injection. Travelers who will arrive in a high-risk area less than 3 weeks from the date of their vaccination should also receive hepatitis immune globulin. A single injection of immune globulin is good for up to 5 months, depending on the dose. Studies have shown that immune globulin prepared in the United States carries no risk of transmission of AIDS. It is also safe to use in pregnancy.

Hepatitis B Vaccine

Although hepatitis B (HB) vaccine was incorporated into the schedule of routine childhood immunizations starting in the late 1980s, HB vaccine is a recommended travel vaccine for certain susceptible adult travelers who are going to areas where the disease is endemic.

Indications

Those who should receive this vaccine include travelers who anticipate exposure to blood or body secretions (e.g., health care personnel, relief workers), unprotected sexual exposure with members of the local population or others, and adventure travel that presents higher risk of accidents and the need for medical attention.

Dosing Schedule for Adults

For adults, the dose of the HB vaccine is 1.0 mL given intramuscularly in the deltoid. The primary immunization schedule consists of three vaccine doses given on a schedule of 0, 1, and 6 months. The vaccine should be given intramuscularly for best response, but hepatitis B vaccine should not be given in the buttock because this route of administration has been associated with a lower immune response.

Accelerated Schedule

The 3-dose primary series may be accelerated to be administered at 0, 1, and 4 or 0, 2, and 4 months, where the second dose is given at least 1 month after the first dose and the third dose is given at least 4 months after the first dose and at 2 months after the second dose.

Japanese Encephalitis Vaccine

Japanese encephalitis (JE) is a mosquito-transmitted virus infection that is endemic in Asia and potentially fatal. In temperate regions the transmission season generally extends from April through November with a peak in July through September. In tropical or subtropical regions of Oceania and Southeast Asia, transmission may occur year-round.

Indications

Decisions regarding the use of JE vaccine for travel must balance the low risk for disease and the small chance of an adverse event following immunization. Consider JE vaccine for travelers who plan to spend a month or longer during the transmission season in endemic areas, particularly in rural areas. Travelers planning extensive unprotected outdoor, evening, and nighttime exposure in rural areas may be at risk even if the trip is very short. Risk of transmission is higher in rural areas, especially where pigs are raised and where rice fields, marshes, and standing pools of water provide breeding grounds for mosquitoes and feed for birds.

Dosing Schedule

For travelers 3 years of age and older, the recommended primary schedule is a series of 3 doses of 1.0 mL of JE-VAX administered by subcutaneous injection on a schedule of 0, 7, and 30 days. The immunity should last for at least 3 years after primary immunization series.

Meningococcal Vaccine

Neisseria meningitidis spreads through the air via droplets of contaminated respiratory secretions, or through person-to-person contact (kissing, sharing cigarettes and drinking glasses, etc.).

Indications

Meningococcal vaccine is recommended for travelers to some countries of Africa during the dry season from December through June, especially if prolonged contact with the local populace is likely. The countries include Benin, Burkina Faso, Cameroon, Central African Republic, Chad, Côte D'Ivoire, Djibouti, Ethiopia, Gambia, Ghana, Guinea, Guinea-Bissau, Mali, Niger, Nigeria, Senegal, Sudan, Somalia, and Togo.

Dosing Schedule for Adults

The quadrivalent meningococcal polysaccharide vaccine consists of a single dose of 0.5 mL by subcutaneous injection to adults. This vaccine should be administered 1 to 2 weeks before departure.

Adverse Events

Minor side effects have been reported, including local pain, swelling, and redness of the skin at the site of injection and, rarely, a low-grade fever.

Rabies Vaccine

Preexposure vaccination against rabies is recommended for travelers to endemic areas who are at increased risk, such as veterinarians, animal handlers, spelunkers, and biologists. A series of three injections over 3 weeks is required.

Typhoid Vaccine

Typhoid fever is an infection transmitted by contaminated food and water. High-risk areas for contracting this illness include Southern Asia; the Middle East; East, West, and Central Africa; and Central and South America. Although an injectable vaccine is still available, the newer oral typhoid vaccine is preferable. Both vaccines protect 50 to 80 percent of recipients.

1. *Typhoid injectable vaccine.* This consists of 2 injections given at least 4 weeks apart. It is good for 3 years. It is about 70 percent effective in preventing the disease and is usually associated with 1 or 2 days of postinjection side effects. These include discomfort at the site of injection, fever, headache, and flulike symptoms.

2. *Oral typhoid vaccine.* This consists of ingesting 4 capsules on alternate days for a total of four capsules over 8 days. A booster is required every 7 years. Adverse reactions are uncommon.

Malaria Vaccine

Malaria is an infection of the bloodstream caused by a parasite transmitted to humans through the bite of the *Anopheles* mosquito. After a period ranging from a week to months, a flulike illness develops, characterized by recurrent fevers, chills, headache, weakness, and lethargy. Fever in a traveler who has returned from a malaria-endemic area should be attributed to malaria until proven otherwise. More than 300 million people are infected each year, with 2 to 3 million deaths; malaria is a significant health threat to travelers.

Prevention

The best way to prevent malaria is to avoid mosquitoes. In Nepal, for example, there is almost no risk in the city of Kathmandu. Traveling to more rural areas increases the risk, and it takes only one bite from an infected mosquito to acquire the disease. The *Anopheles* mosquito feeds at night. Thus, maximum precautions should be taken from dusk to dawn. One should wear thin, loose clothing that covers the arms and legs. At dusk, tuck pants into socks or shoes, and tape the cuffs of shirt sleeves closed. Use screens, mosquito nets, and repellents at night. The most effective repellents contain 35 to 50 percent DEET (N, N-diethyltoluamide). Studies suggest that concentrations of DEET above 50 percent do not offer a marked increase in protection against mosquitoes. The duration of action is between 2 to 6 hours, depending on the concentration of DEET, how much the wearer perspires, and how hungry the mosquito is. Rare case reports of adverse reactions to

DEET range from skin rashes to central nervous system (brain) disorders. Spraying or soaking clothing and bed nets with permethrin and letting them air-dry before use is also very helpful.

Antimalarial Drugs for Prevention

All recommended malaria-prevention regimens involve taking a medicine before travel, during travel, and for a period of time after leaving the malaria-endemic area. Beginning the drug before travel allows the antimalarial agent to be in the blood before the traveler is exposed to malaria parasites and to observe for any adverse reactions. No antimalarial drug is absolutely effective. A traveler can still develop the disease regardless of how many medications are taken.

Tools such as the interactive malaria map (www.cdc.gov/malaria /map) can assist in locating specific countries where malaria protection is needed. Updated information can be obtained by referring to the *CDC Health Information for International Travel* (The Yellow Book), or the online version at the CDC Travelers' Health website (wwwnc.cdc .gov/travel), or by calling the CDC Malaria Hotline by phone: 770-488-7788. Information on diagnosis and treatment of malaria is also available online (www.cdc.gov/malaria).

Chloroquine

In only a few places in the world is chloroquine still effective in preventing malaria. Chloroquine is recommended for travel to Central America west of the Panama Canal Zone, Mexico, Haiti, the Dominican Republic, Egypt, and most countries in the Middle East (chloroquine resistance has been reported in Iran, Yemen, and Oman). The drug is generally safe, but side effects can include nausea, diarrhea, and upset stomach. It is taken once weekly, beginning 2 weeks prior to departure, continued weekly during travel in malarious areas, and for 4 weeks after leaving such areas.

Mefloquine

Mefloquine is now the most widely prescribed drug for the prevention of malaria in parts of the world where the parasite is resistant to chloroquine. The adult dose is 250 mg once a week. The pediatric dose varies according to the weight of the child. Check with a pediatrician.

Mefloquine should be started 1 to 2 weeks before travel and contin-ued for 4 weeks after leaving the endemic area. Mefloquine should not be taken during pregnancy, or if on a beta-blocker or calcium channel blocker medication.

Mefloquine can occasionally produce serious adverse reactions, such as acute psychoses, hallucinations, anxiety, and seizures. Other side effects include nausea, upset stomach, and diarrhea.

Doxycycline

An alternative to mefloquine is doxycycline 100 mg daily, beginning 1 to 2 days before travel to malarious areas. This drug is not advised for pregnant women or children under 8 years of age. It can also cause a rash in users exposed to the sun. (Vaccination with the oral typhoid vaccine should be delayed for at least 24 hours after taking a dose of doxycycline.)

Proguanil (Paludrine)

This drug may be used for malaria prevention where there is resis-tance to chloroquine. The adult dose is 200 mg daily along with weekly chloroquine.

Atovaquone and Proguanil (Malarone)

Atovaquone in combination with proguanil is available as the drug Malarone and can be taken to prevent chloroquine-resistant malaria. The drug is taken at the same time each day with food or a milky drink. The drug should be started 2 days before entering a malaria-endemic area and continued for 7 days after return. The adult dose is 1 tablet (250 mL atovaquone/100 mg proguanil) per day. Malarone is very well tolerated, and side effects are rare. The most common adverse effects are abdominal pain, nausea, and headache.

Pyrimethamine and Sulfadoxine (Fansidar)

Fansidar is a combination drug containing pyrimethamine and sul-fadoxine. Because of the drug's association with an unacceptably high incidence of toxic side effects when used for prevention, it is generally reserved only for treatment.

Latent Malaria

Certain forms of malaria *(Plasmodium vivax)* can hide in the liver and cause illness for as long as 4 years after returning from an endemic country. The drug primaquine, taken after the traveler has left a malaria area, can prevent this from occurring.

Treatment of Malaria

Malaria can be treated effectively early in the course of the disease, but delay of therapy can have serious or fatal consequences. Travelers who have symptoms of malaria should seek medical evaluation as soon as possible. CDC recommendations for malaria treatment can be found online (www.cdc.gov/malaria/diagnosis_treatment).

Consider self-treatment for a traveler who develops symptoms of malaria (fever, chills, and other flulike symptoms) in a malaria-endemic area while not taking prophylactic malaria medicine, or those who chose a suboptimal drug regimen (e.g., chloroquine in an area with chloroquine-resistant malaria). Consider atovaquone/proguanil (Malarone) for self-treatment if professional medical care is not available within 24 hours. Medical care should be sought immediately after treatment. The adult dose is 4 tablets (each dose contains 1000 mg atovaquone and 400 mg proguanil) orally as a single daily dose for 3 consecutive days.

Medical Advice and Assistance

The International Association for Medical Assistance to Travellers (IAMAT), established in 1960, is a voluntary organization of hospitals, health care centers, and physicians. Its volunteers include more than 3000 English-speaking, Western-trained doctors in over 140 countries. All fees are standardized. Each year, the IAMAT publishes an updated directory of its member physicians as well as pamphlets on immunization requirements, climate, malaria, and schistosomiasis. IAMAT membership is free. In the United States, contact IAMAT at 1623 Military Rd. #279, Niagara Falls, NY 14304-1745, 716-754-4883, www.iamat.org.

OTHER COMMON TRAVEL DISEASES

Typhoid Fever

Typhoid fever is a common disease caused by a bacterium *(Salmonella typhi)* and transmitted by ingestion of food or water contaminated with the feces of an infected person.

Signs and Symptoms

Symptoms usually begin 10 to 14 days after exposure to the bacteria. Fever is usually the first sign of disease. Headache, fatigue, abdominal cramps, diarrhea or constipation, and dizziness often occur. A red rash that blanches with pressure sometimes develops on the trunk.

Treatment

Most victims get better on their own after 3 to 4 weeks. A few individuals will develop severe complications, including intestinal perforation and peritonitis. Antibiotics (ampicillin or ciprofloxacin [Cipro]) can be used to treat the illness.

Dengue Fever

Dengue fever is a very common mosquito-transmitted viral infection. It is now endemic in Asia, the South Pacific, the Caribbean basin, Mexico, Central America, South America, and Africa.

Signs and Symptoms

Dengue fever is characterized by sudden onset of high fever, severe frontal headache, and joint and muscle pains, which can be so painful that the illness is sometimes called "breakbone fever." Many victims have nausea and vomiting, and develop a rash 3 to 5 days after onset of fever. The symptoms can be similar to and even mistaken for malaria.

Treatment

The illness is usually self-limited and lasts about a week. Occasionally, a victim will remain very weak for up to a month or will develop a severe and fatal syndrome called dengue hemorrhagic fever. There is no specific treatment, and a vaccine is not available.

Schistosomiasis

Schistosomiasis is a parasitic disease transmitted by freshwater snails that excrete the parasite into freshwater ponds, lakes, or rivers. The parasite then penetrates the skin of humans during bathing or swimming in infested water. The countries where schistosomiasis is most common include Brazil, Egypt, sub-Saharan Africa, southern China, the Philippines, and Southeast Asia.

Signs and Symptoms

Symptoms usually start 2 to 3 weeks after exposure and include fever, loss of appetite, abdominal pain, weakness, headaches, joint and muscle pain, diarrhea, nausea, cough, and itchy rash. Infection of the brain can produce seizures and visual loss.

Treatment

Praziquantel (Biltricide), an antiparasitic drug, will effectively cure the illness.

West Nile Virus

Mosquitoes transmit this virus, and birds are the most common reservoir.

Signs and Symptoms

The incubation period from bite to infection is 3 to 14 days. Most infections are asymptomatic or present with mild flulike illness. Severe infections include meningitis and encephalitis.

Treatment

No specific treatment is available. Therapy is supportive.

Leptospirosis

Leptospirosis is caused by a spirochete that enters the body though the skin, eyes, mouth, or nose during swimming or bathing in fresh water. Thus, activities that are likely to lead to infection include rafting, kayaking, or swimming in fresh water where the disease is endemic.

Signs and Symptoms

After an incubation period of 7 to 12 days, the victim develops high fever, headache, chills, muscle aches, and red eyes without exudate. After a few days, the victim seems to recover, only to develop the return of less dramatic fever associated with relentless headache, and possibly jaundice and a red rash.

Treatment

The treatment of choice is doxycycline 100 mg twice daily for 7 days. Tetracycline 2 g in four divided doses for 7 to 14 days is an alternative.

Malaria
(See "Malaria Vaccine," page 188.)

Cutaneous Myiasis (Botfly Infection)

Botfly (*Dermatobia hominis*) infections are common in travelers to the jungles of Central and South America. The female fly attaches her eggs to the body of another arthropod (usually a mosquito), which then transfers the egg to the skin of a human when it lands for a meal. The eggs hatch immediately, and the larvae crawl into the skin through the bite wound, where they continue to grow.

Signs and Symptoms

Initially the wound looks and feels like another mosquito bite. The victim is eventually alerted that something else is going on when the bump gets larger over time and becomes quite painful. A sensation of movement may be felt within the bump. A characteristic central opening (breathing hole) drains clear fluid when the bump is squeezed. The developing larvae just underneath the skin can be mistaken for a bacteria-infected bite, leading to unnecessary antibiotics or, worse, incision and drainage.

Treatment

First, cover the opening with DEET-containing repellent or permethrin and wait about 30 minutes for it to kill the larvae. When the larvae die they release their attachment to the skin. Then forcefully squeeze the skin adjacent to the bump to extrude the larvae.

:bulb: Weiss Advice

Smoking Out Botfly Larvae

Blowing cigarette smoke onto your hand will create a lethal deposit of nicotine, which can then be transferred to the bump and smeared over the hole. Leave it in place for 20 to 30 minutes before squeezing. Duct tape, smeared with petroleum jelly or nail polish remover, will also suffocate the larvae if placed tightly over the hole.

Motion Sickness

Air, ocean, and bumpy bus travel are often associated with motion sickness. It is caused by fluid movement in the inner ear.

Signs and Symptoms

Symptoms include pale skin, sweating, nausea, and weakness. These symptoms are usually made worse by alcohol ingestion, emotional upset, noxious odors, and ear infections. Symptoms will not dissipate until the inner ear has had a chance to acclimate to motion (usually within a few days) or is treated with medication.

Treatment

To control motion sickness, first try fixing your eyes on a steady point in the distance. Move to the center of the plane, boat, or bus, where motion is minimized. If particularly prone to motion sickness, you can try taking meclizine (Antivert) 25 mg orally or dimenhydrinate (Dramamine) 50 mg orally every 6 to 12 hours, beginning 2 to 3 hours before travel. Diphenhydramine (Benadryl) has also been shown to help prevent and treat motion sickness. For the medication to be most effective, it should be started before encountering a situation that can lead to motion sickness.

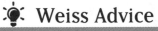

☀ Weiss Advice

Curbing Motion Sickness with Ginger

Ginger root has been shown to be very effective in curbing the nausea caused by motion sickness. Ginger is ordinarily taken in the form of capsules, each containing 500 mg of the powdered herb. The average recommended daily dose is 2 to 3 grams. It may also be consumed as a tea or in the extract form. There are no reports of severe toxicity in humans from eating recommended amounts of ginger.

Jet Lag

Jet lag is common among travelers who cross several time zones. While the symptoms are usually mild, it can be difficult for a person to function until the body's rhythms have had a chance to adjust.

Signs and Symptoms

Symptoms include irritability, insomnia, headache, loss of appetite, and a general feeling of malaise. Dehydration, which commonly occurs on long flights, may be a factor in the severity of jet lag.

Treatment

Drinking fluids and avoiding alcohol until adjusted to the new time zone can be very helpful. A low dose of a short-acting sleeping pill such as zolpidem (Ambien) 5–10 mg can be taken for the first 2 to 3 nights after arrival to facilitate sleep.

Exposure to bright light for 5 to 7 hours a day for 2 to 3 days may help reset one's internal clock. Travelers going eastward should expose themselves to bright light in the early morning, while those traveling westward should expose themselves to bright light in the late afternoon.

The hormone melatonin—5 mg taken at bedtime for 2 days before travel, then for 3 days after arrival—may also help reset the body's internal clock. Little, however, is known about the long-term safety of melatonin. It should not be taken by children; women who are pregnant, nursing, or trying to conceive; or people with cancer, severe allergies, or on steroid therapy.

WATER DISINFECTION

There are three proven techniques for removing infectious organisms (bacteria, viruses, and parasites) from water: filters, boiling, and chemical treatment.

WATER FILTERS

Filters are commercially available with pore sizes small enough to remove Giardia organisms and most bacteria from water. Many now also have iodine resins, which can kill viruses (see below).

BOILING WATER

Much of the time required to bring water to a boil works toward disinfecting it. By the time water reaches its boiling point, the water is safe to drink. Although the boiling point of water decreases with altitude, this does not make a difference, since almost all organisms are killed well below the boiling point of water.

CHEMICAL DISINFECTION

The two most common chemicals used to disinfect water are chlorine and iodine. Iodine is preferred over chlorine in the backcountry for several reasons:

1. Iodine is less affected by pH and nitrogenous wastes.
2. Iodine imparts a taste that is better tolerated than that of chlorine.
3. Iodine is easier to transport.
4. Iodine can double as a topical disinfectant for wound care.

Iodine will not kill Cryptosporidium at concentrations used for disinfecting drinking water. To kill Giardia, iodine must be allowed to sit in the water for a longer time.

Iodine takes longer to work in cold water, so the dose or the contact time with the water must be increased. Some iodine is absorbed by impurities in the water, so more iodine is required for cloudy or polluted water. Add flavoring to the water, if you wish, but only after the iodine has had adequate contact time with the water.

Table 3
10% Povidone-Iodine Solution (Betadine)
Measure with dropper (1 drop = 0.05 mL)
Add to 1 liter or quart of water

Drops per Liter or Quart	Water Temperature	Water Clarity	Contact Time
8	Warm	Clear	30 min.
16	Warm	Cloudy	30 min.
8	Cold	Clear	60 min.
16	Cold	Cloudy	60 min.
	Less than 10°C/50°F		

Iodine Tablets

Tablets per Liter or Quart	Water Temperature	Water Clarity	Contact Time
1	Warm	Clear	15 min.
2	Warm	Cloudy	15 min.
1	Cold	Clear	45 min.
2	Cold	Cloudy	45 min.

Source: Data from H.D. Backer, *"Field Water Disinfection," Wilderness Medicine: Management of Wilderness and Environmental Emergencies*, 3rd edition. Ed. P.S. Auerbach (Mosby, 1995).

Liquid household bleach (sodium hypochlorite, usually 5.25–6.15%) can be used to disinfect water via chlorination (see the following table). Filter the liquid through a water purifier or coffee filter to remove any solid impurities. A faint smell or taste of chlorine should be detectable before drinking.

Table 4
Sodium Hypochlorite (Bleach)

Drops per Liter or Quart	Water Temperature	Water Clarity	Contact Time
2	Warm	Clear	30 min
4	Warm	Cloudy	30 min
2	Cold	Clear	60 min
4	Cold	Cloudy	60 min
	Note· Warm water is >15°C (60°F).		

WILDERNESS FIRST-AID KITS

When designing a wilderness first-aid kit, several prerequisites and variables are important to consider:

- Your medical expertise
- The location and environmental extremes of your destination
- Diseases that may be particular to an area of travel
- The duration of travel
- Your distance from definitive medical care and the availability of professional rescue
- The number of people the kit will need to support
- Preexisting illnesses that someone may have
- Weight and space limitations

The wilderness medical kit should be well organized in a protective and convenient carrying pouch. For backpacking, trekking, or hiking, a nylon organizer bag is optimal. Newer-generation bags with clear, protective compartments have proven superior to mesh-covered pockets. The clear cover, protects the components from dirt, moisture, and insects, and prevents items from falling out when the kit is turned on its side or upside down. Look for organizer bags with clearly marked pockets separating the items by injury so you can quickly find what you need in an emergency.

For aquatic environments, the kit should be stored in a waterproof dry bag or watertight hard container. Inside, items should be sealed in zipper-lock bags, since moisture will invariably make its way into any container.

Some medicines may need to be stored outside of the main kit to ensure protection from extreme temperatures. For example, capsules and suppositories melt when exposed to body temperature heat (37°C [98.6°F]), and many liquid medicines become useless after freezing.

GENERAL EQUIPMENT
- Accident report form
- **Bandage scissors**. Designed with a blunt tip to protect the patient while cutting through clothes, boots, or bandages.
- **Cotton-tipped applicators**. May be used to remove insects or other foreign material from the eye. Also useful to roll fluid out from beneath a blister, or to evert an eyelid to locate a foreign body.
- **CPR Face Shield**. Compact and easy-to-use, clear, flexible barriers for performing mouth-to-mouth rescue breathing. Prevents physical contact with the victim's secretions.
- Duct tape
- **Glutose paste**. Oral glucose gel containing concentrated sugar for treating hypoglycemia and insulin reactions in diabetics, and for hypothermia.
- **Hypothermia (low reading) thermometers**. Ideally should be able to read temperatures from 30 to 40°C (85 to 107°F).
- Pencil and paper
- Plastic resealable (zipper-lock) bags
- Safety pins
- **C-Splint**. A 10 x 91-cm (4 x 36-inch) foam-padded aluminum splint. Adaptable for use on almost any part of the body, it can be fashioned as cervical collar or arm, leg, or ankle splint.

WOUND MANAGEMENT
- **0.5 x 10-cm (¼ x 4-inch) wound closure strips**. These are excellent for closing cuts in the wilderness. Wound closure strips are stronger, longer, stickier, and more porous than the common butterfly-type adhesive bandages.
- **10- to 20-cc irrigation syringe** with an 18-gauge catheter tip. Using the syringe like a squirt gun flushes out germs from wounds without harming the delicate tissues.
- **Forceps or tweezers**. For removing embedded objects from the skin, such as splinters, cactus thorns, ticks, or stingers.
- **Nitrile barrier gloves**. To protect the rescuer from infectious diseases such as hepatitis and AIDS. Latex gloves can cause serious allergic reactions and should be avoided.

> ▓ **Surgical scrub brush.** A sterile scrub brush for cleaning embedded objects and dirt from abrasions.

TOPICAL TREATMENTS

> ▓ **Aloe vera gel.** A topical anti-inflammatory for treating burns, frostbite, abrasions, poison oak, and poison ivy.
> ▓ **Antiseptic towelettes with benzalkonium chloride.** Disposable wipes that may be used to clean wounds. Benzalkonium chloride may help to kill the rabies virus on wounds inflicted by animals.
> ▓ **Antibiotic ointment.** A topical antibiotic ointment that helps to prevent minor skin infections and accelerates wound healing. Avoid triple antibiotic ointments that contain neomycin as they can produce an allergic rash in susceptible individuals.
> ▓ **Povidone-iodine solution USP 10% (Betadine).** To disinfect backcountry water and to sterilize wound edges. When diluted ten-fold with water, the solution can be used for wound irrigation.
> ▓ **Topical skin adhesive.** A liquid adhesive, containing either tincture of benzoin or rosin, that enhances the stickiness of wound closure strips or tape.
> ▓ **Alcohol wipes.** To clean and dry area around the wound before applying tape or moleskin. Allows better skin adhesion.

BANDAGE MATERIAL

> ▓ 10 x 10-cm (4 x 4-inch), 8 x 8-cm (3 x 3-inch), or 5 x 5-cm (2 x 2-inch) sterile dressings
> ▓ 20 x 25-cm (8 x 10-inch) or 13 x 23-cm (5 x 9-inch) sterile trauma pads
> ▓ Assortment of strip and knuckle adhesive bandages
> ▓ **Elastic roll bandage** (e.g., ACE wrap). Used to hold dressings in place or to create a pressure bandage for bleeding or for sprains.
> ▓ **Gauze roller bandages** (e.g., Kling). A bandage that is used to keep the dressing in place and further protect a wound from the environment.
> ▓ **Molefoam.** A thick, padded adhesive material for protecting blisters. Cut a doughnut shape out of the material and place it around a blister site.

- **Moleskin.** A thin, padded adhesive material for protecting skin from developing blisters. Adventure Medical Kit's precut and shaped moleskin pieces are easy to apply and do not require scissors to use. They can be layered to provide a raised area to protect already developed blisters.
- **GlacierGel Blister and Burn Dressings.** 50% water-based gel dressings on a waterproof and breathable adhesive film. Easy to apply and lasts up to 4 days. GlacierGel dressings eliminate pain from blisters and burns. Clear gel dressings allow you to monitor the blister or burn site for infection.
- **Nonadherent sterile dressings.** Nonstick dressings that are used to cover abrasions, burns, lacerations, and blisters. Some examples include GlacierGel, Aquaphor, Xeroform, Adaptic, and Telfa.
- **Stockinette bandage.** A net-style bandage particularly useful for holding dressings in place across a joint.
- **Surgical (cloth or paper) tape**
- **Triangular bandage.** Useful for making a sling and swath, holding splints in place, or improvising a foot harness for a traction splint.

NONPRESCRIPTION MEDICATIONS FOR BASIC FIRST-AID KIT

WARNING: A physician should be consulted before any medication is taken by a child, pregnant woman, or nursing mother. Make sure recipients are not allergic to any drugs you plan to administer. Sharing medications with others is potentially hazardous and is not recommended. Read the instructions carefully on the medication package, and do not use it if you think the recipient may be allergic to the drug.

Acetaminophen (Tylenol)

Indications. For relief of pain and fever. Acetaminophen (Tylenol) has no anti-inflammatory effect.

Dosage. *Adults:* Take two 325 mg. tablets every 4-6 hours. Do not take more than 12 tablets in 24 hours. *Children 6-11 year-old:* 1 tablet every 4-6 hours. Do not take more than 5 tablets in 24 hours. *Under 6:* consult a pediatrician.

WARNING: In case of overdose, contact a physician or poison control center immediately. Individuals with liver disease, and those who regularly consume alcohol or are allergic to this medicine, should not use this.

Aloe Vera Gel

Indications. A topical treatment for first-degree and second-degree burns, frostbite, abrasions, and blisters.

Dosage. Apply a thin coat to the affected area two to three times a day.

WARNING: Discontinue use if redness, swelling, or pain develops at the site.

Aluminum Hydroxide and Simethicone (Mylanta)

Indications. Each tablet contains both an antacid and an anti-gas ingredient. Helps relieve heartburn, acid indigestion, sour stomach, and gas. Provides symptomatic relief of peptic ulcer disease and gastritis.

Dosage. 2 to 4 tablets between meals and at bedtime.

WARNING: Individuals who have kidney disease should not use this drug. It can interfere with the absorption of certain antibiotics. If symptoms persist, consult a physician as soon as possible.

Diphenhydramine (Benadryl)

Indications. An antihistamine that can temporarily relieve runny nose, sneezing, watery eyes, and itchy throat due to hay fever or other respiratory allergies and colds. Relieves itching and rash associated with allergic reactions, including poison oak or poison ivy. Useful as an adjunct to epinephrine in the treatment of severe allergic shock. May also prevent and help relieve the symptoms of motion sickness.

Dosage. Adults: 25 to 50 mg every 4 to 6 hours. *Children*: Consult your physician.

WARNING: May cause drowsiness. Individuals with asthma, glaucoma, high blood pressure, emphysema, or prostatic enlargement should not use this drug unless directed to do so by a physician. Not recommended for use in hot environments, when heat illness is likely, during pregnancy, or while taking other anticholinergic medications. (Consult physician before use.)

Hydrocortisone Cream USP 1%

Indications. For temporary relief of minor skin irritations and allergic reactions.

Dosage. Adults and children 2 years of age and older: Apply to affected area not more than three to four times a day. *Children under 2 years*: Consult a physician.

WARNING: If condition worsens or if symptoms persist for more than 7 days or clear up and occur again within a few days, stop use of this product and do not begin use of any other hydrocortisone product unless you have consulted a physician. Do not use for the treatment of diaper rash. In case of accidental ingestion, seek professional assistance or contact a poison control center immediately. Keep this and all drugs out of the reach of children. For external use only. Avoid contact with eyes.

Ibuprofen (Motrin)

Indications. For the temporary relief of minor aches and pains associated with the common cold, headache, toothache, muscular aches, backache, and arthritis. Also effective in reducing the inflammation associated with sprains, strains, bursitis, tendonitis, minor burns, and frostbite. Reduces the pain of menstrual cramps and lowers fever.

Dosage. *Adults*: 400 to 800 mg every 8 hours with food. Do not take on an empty stomach. *Children*: Ibuprofen is available by prescription in liquid form for children.

WARNING: It may cause upset stomach or heartburn. Individuals who are allergic to aspirin or any other nonsteroidal anti-inflammatory drug should not take this drug. Individuals who have kidney disease, have gastritis, have ulcers, are prone to bleeding, or are on any blood thinner medication should not take it. It is not recommended for use during pregnancy.

Oral Rehydration Salt Packets (Electrolyte Salts and Glucose)

When combined with a liter or quart of water, these packets provide an ideal solution for replacing electrolytes and fluids lost during diarrhea illness, heat exhaustion, or vomiting.

Bismuth Subsalicylate (Pepto-Bismol)

Each tablet contains 262 mg bismuth subsalicylate.

Indications. May prevent and help treat traveler's diarrhea, nausea, and upset stomach.

Dosage. 2 tablets four times a day.

WARNING: Individuals allergic to aspirin should not use this medication. Children and teenagers who have or are recovering from chicken pox or flu should not use this medication to treat vomiting. If vomiting occurs, consult a physician as this could be an early sign of Reye's syndrome, a rare but serious illness. As with any drug, if you are pregnant or nursing a baby, seek the advice of a health professional before using.

RECOMMENDED PRESCRIPTION MEDICATIONS FOR ADVANCED FIRST-AID KIT

WARNING: A physician should be consulted before any medication is taken by a child, pregnant woman, or nursing mother. Make sure recipients are not allergic to any drugs that you plan to administer. Sharing medications with others is potentially hazardous and is not recommended. Do not treat yourself or others unless there is no alternative and you are comfortable with the problem. Dosages differ for adults and children; unless otherwise specified, dosages listed here are for adults. Carefully review the dose, indications, and adverse effects of all drugs that you plan to carry.

EPINEPHRINE AUTO-INJECTORS (EPIPEN AND EPIPEN JR)

Epinephrine quickly constricts blood vessels and relaxes smooth muscles. It improves breathing, stimulates the heart to beat faster and harder, and relieves hives and swelling.

Indications. Emergency treatment of severe allergic reactions (anaphylaxis) to bees, wasps, hornets, yellow jackets, foods, drugs, and other allergens. May also help relieve symptoms of asthma.

Dosage. Adults and children over 30 kg (66 pounds): Each EpiPen contains 2 mL of epinephrine 1:1000 USP in a disposable push-button spring-activated cartridge with a concealed needle. It will deliver a single dose of 0.3 mg epinephrine intramuscularly. Swing and firmly push the orange tip against the outer thigh so it "clicks." HOLD on thigh for approximately 10 seconds to deliver the drug. As soon as you release pressure from the thigh, the protective cover will extend. The drug should be felt within 1 to 2 minutes. *Children who weigh less than 30 kg (66 pounds)*: The EpiPen Jr will deliver a single dose of 0.15 mg of epinephrine.

WARNING: Unless the situation is life-threatening, epinephrine should be avoided in individuals who are 50 years old and older or have a known heart condition. Sometimes a single dose of epinephrine may not be enough to completely reverse the effects of an anaphylactic reaction. For individuals who know they have severe allergic reactions, it may be wise to carry more than one auto-injector.

ANTIBIOTICS

Some of the antibiotics listed below have similar uses and overlapping spectrums of antibacterial activity. Before departing on your trip, discuss with your physician which antibiotics best suit your needs.

Amoxicillin Clavulanate (Augmentin) 500 mg Tablets

A broad-spectrum penicillin-type antibiotic.

Indications. Bite wounds, skin infections, pneumonia, urinary tract infections, ear infections, bronchitis, tonsillitis, sinusitis.

Dosage. 1 tablet every 8 hours, for 7 to 10 days.

WARNING: Do not use if allergic to penicillin. Stop use if rash develops. May cause diarrhea.

Azithromycin (Zithromax) 250 mg Capsules

A broad-spectrum, erythromycin-type antibiotic. It is more potent than erythromycin, causes fewer side effects, and only has to be taken once a day for 5 days.

Indications. Tonsillitis, ear infections, bronchitis, pneumonia, sinusitis, traveler's diarrhea, skin infections.

Dosage. Take 2 capsules on the first day, followed by 1 capsule a day for 4 more days.

WARNING: Individuals who are allergic to erythromycin should not use azithromycin. Do not use simultaneously with the antihistamines terfenadine (Seldane) or astemizote (Hismanal).

Cefuroxime (Ceftin) or Cephalexin (Keflex) 250 to 500 mg Tablets

Broad-spectrum antibiotics, which can be substituted for amoxicillin clavulanate (Augmentin) in individuals allergic to penicillin.

Indications. Skin infections, bronchitis, urinary tract infections, tonsillitis, middle ear infections, some bone infections, bite wounds, dental infections, sinusitis.

Dosage. 250–500 mg every 6 hours.

WARNING: Avoid or use with caution in individuals with penicillin allergy, since 5 percent of people may be cross-reactive.

Ciprofloxacin (Cipro) 500 mg Tablets

An excellent antibiotic for traveler's diarrhea and dysentery.

Indications. Diarrhea, pneumonia, urinary tract infections, bone infections.

Dosage. 1 tablet twice a day for 3 days. For kidney infections, pneumonia, and bone infections, treat for 7 to 10 days.

WARNING: Not recommended for patients less than 18 years old or pregnant or nursing women. Adverse effects, although uncommon, have included nausea, vomiting, diarrhea, and abdominal pain.

Polymyxin B Sulfates and Neomycin with Hydrocortisone (Cortisporin Otic Suspension)

Indications. External ear infections (swimmer's ear).

Dosage. 4 drops instilled into the affected ear four times a day.

WARNING: Discontinue using if a rash develops or the condition worsens.

Erythromycin 250/500 mg Tablets

An alternative antibiotic for individuals allergic to penicillin.

Indications. Bronchitis, tonsillitis, pneumonia, skin infections, sinus infections, ear and eye infections.

Dosage. 250–500 mg every 6 hours for 7 to 10 days.

WARNING: May cause upset stomach, vomiting, and/or diarrhea. Take with food.

Levofloxacin (Levaquin) 500 mg Tablets

Indications. Bronchitis, pneumonia, urinary tract infections, sinusitis, skin infections, anthrax.

Dosage. 500 mg every 24 hours for 7 to 14 days.

WARNING: Fluoroquinolones, including levofloxacin (Levaquin), are associated with an increased risk of tendinitis and tendon rupture in all ages.

Metronidazole (Flagyl) 250 mg Tablets

Indications. Intra-abdominal infections including peritonitis and appendicitis, dental infections.

Dosage. Intra-abdominal infections: 2 tablets every 6 hours if the patient is not vomiting.

WARNING: Do not drink alcohol while taking this medication. The interaction will cause severe abdominal pain, nausea, and vomiting. May cause unpleasant metallic taste. Do not use during pregnancy.

Nitazoxanide (Alinia) 500 mg Tablets

Indications. Giardiasis and cryptosporidiosis.

Dosage. *Adults*: 500 mg twice a day for 3 days. *Children*: 100 mg twice a day for 3 days.

Trimethoprim/Sulfamethoxazole (Septra DS or Bactrim DS)

Each tablet contains 80 mg trimethoprim and 400 mg sulfamethoxazole.

Indications. Urinary tract or kidney infections, ear and sinus infections, bronchitis. Recommended for skin infections when methicillin-resistant *Staphylococcus aureus* (MRSA) might be the source of the infection.

Dosage. 1 tablet twice a day for 5 days for diarrhea and dysentery. Other infections may require a 10-day course.

WARNING: Individuals allergic to sulfa drugs should not use this drug. Trimethoprim 200 mg alone, twice a day, may be substituted for treatment of diarrhea and dysentery. Discontinue use at the first sign of skin rash or any adverse reaction. Do not use during pregnancy.

FOR NAUSEA AND VOMITING

Prochlorperazine (Compazine) or Promethazine (Phenergan) Suppositories

Indications. For control of severe nausea and vomiting.

Dosage. 25 mg rectally twice a day.

WARNING: *Do not use in children*. Side effects include neck spasm, difficulty in swallowing and talking, sensation that the tongue is thick, muscle stiffness, and agitation. If these symptoms occur, discontinue use of the drug and administer diphenhydramine (Benadryl) 50 mg. May produce drowsiness.

Ondansetron (Zofran ODT) 4 mg

Indications. For control of severe nausea and vomiting.

Dosage. Place 4 mg tablet on tongue immediately after opening blister pack and allow it to dissolve. Handle with dry hands. Do not cut or chew tablet.

SYMPTOMATIC RELIEF OF DIARRHEA

Loperamide (Imodium) 2 mg Capsule

(Also available over the counter)

Indications. For controlling the abdominal cramping and diarrhea associated with intestinal infections.

Dosage. 4 mg initially, followed by 1 capsule (2 mg) after each loose bowel movement not to exceed 14 mg in one day.

WARNING: Imodium should not be used if there is associated fever (greater than 38°C [101°F], blood or pus in the stool, or swollen abdomen. It should not be used for more than 48 hours. *This drug should not be given to children.*

EYE INFECTIONS

Tobramycin (Tobrex) Ophthalmic Solution 0.3%

A topical antibiotic for the eye.

Indications. For external infections of the eye (conjunctivitis or pinkeye, or corneal abrasions).

Dosage. 1 to 2 drops into the affected eye every 2 hours while awake.

WARNING: Individuals who develop or have an allergy or sensitivity to this medicine should not use it.

PAIN MEDICATION

Acetaminophen with Hydrocodone (Vicodin)

Each tablet contains hydrocodone 5 mg and acetaminophen 500 mg.

Indications. For relief of pain. Can also be used for relief of diarrhea and suppression of coughs.

Dosage. 1 to 2 tablets every 4 to 6 hours.

WARNING: Codeine is a narcotic and may be habit-forming. Side effects include drowsiness, respiratory depression, constipation, and nausea. Individuals who are allergic to either acetaminophen or codeine should not use this medication.

ALTITUDE ILLNESS

Acetazolamide (Diamox) 250 mg Tablets

Indications. May help to prevent altitude illness when used in conjunction with graded ascent and to treat altitude illness in conjunction with descent. Useful in diminishing the sleep disorder associated with mountain sickness.

Dosage. For prevention, 125 mg ($^1/_2$ tablet) twice a day, beginning the day before the ascent. For treatment, 250 mg twice a day until symptoms resolve.

WARNING: Acetazolamide (Diamox) is not a substitute for graded ascent and acclimatization, nor a substitute for descent in the event of severe altitude illness. Side effects include increased urination, numbness in the fingers and toes, and lethargy. Carbonated beverages will also taste terrible. Do not use if allergic to sulfa medications.

Dexamethasone (Decadron)

Indications. For the treatment of high-altitude cerebral edema (HACE) in conjunction with immediate descent to a lower altitude. For prevention of acute mountain sickness when rapid ascent is required.

Dosage. 8 mg initially, followed by 4 mg every 6 hours.

Nifedipine (Procardia)

Indications. For the treatment of high-altitude pulmonary edema (HAPE) in conjunction with immediate descent to a lower altitude.

Dosage. 10 mg every 4 hours, or 10 mg one time followed by 30 mg extended-release capsule every 12 to 24 hours.

WARNING: May cause low blood pressure and fainting, especially when standing up from a lying position.

BASIC DENTAL KIT

- ▓ Cavit temporary filling material
- ▓ Cotton pellets
- ▓ Cotton rolls
- ▓ Dental floss
- ▓ Eugenol (oil of cloves)
- ▓ Zinc oxide. Mixing together zinc oxide and eugenol will make a temporary filling, which sets in a few minutes after contact with saliva

MEDICAL SUPPLIES FOR EXTENDED EXPEDITIONS AND SPECIAL ENVIRONMENTS

- Advanced Wound Management Supplies
- 1% lidocaine hydrochloride (Xylocaine) for anesthesia
- Surgical staples
- Suture set and suture material
- Airway supplies (oral or nasal airways, endotracheal and crico-thyrodotomy tubes)
- Foley catheter
- Intravenous solutions and administration tubing
- Needles and syringes
- Urine Chemstrips for diagnosing urinary tract infections
- Urine pregnancy test

Marine Environment
- 5% acetic acid (vinegar)
- Prednisone

Cold Environment
- Glutose paste (concentrated sugar to help the body generate heat)
- Low-reading (down to at least 30°C [85°F]) thermometer
- Matches

Jungle or Developing World Travel
- Antibiotics for treating traveler's diarrhea—ciprofloxacin (Cipro) or azithromycin (Zithromax)
- Clotrimazole and betamethasone dipropionate cream (Lotrisone) for treating fungal infections
- Insect repellent
- Loperamide (Imodium) for symptomatic relief of diarrhea
- Oral rehydration salt packets
- Permethrin 5% cream and 1% shampoo for treating lice, bed-bugs, and scabies

INTERNET INFORMATION RESOURCES FOR WILDERNESS AND FOREIGN TRAVELERS

The American Society of Tropical Medicine and Hygiene (ASTMH): Worldwide community of researchers, clinicians, and professionals dedicated to advancing global health through collaboration, education, and career advancement in tropical medicine. www.astmh.org/source/ClinicalDirectory

Centers for Disease Control and Prevention (CDC): Travel health information to address the many different health risks a traveler may face, including (1) *broad-based travelers' health information*, including destinations, diseases, vaccinations, illness and injury abroad, finding a clinic, how to stay healthy (wwwnc.cdc.gov/travel); (2) *Center for Global Health*, coordinates and manages collective resources and expertise to address a variety of global health challenges, such as HIV/AIDS, malaria, emergency and refugee health, noncommunicable diseases, injuries, and other health threats (www.cdc.gov/globalhealth); (3) *resources about malaria* (www.cdc.gov/malaria, www.cdc.gov/malaria/diagnosis_treatment, www.cdc.gov/malaria/map); (4) *The Yellow Book*, published every 2 years by CDC as a reference for those who advise international travelers about health risks, written primarily for health professionals, although others will find it useful (wwwnc/cdc.gov/travel/page/yellowbook-2012-home.htm); (5) *resources about tickborne diseases of the U.S. (www.cdc.gov/ticks/diseases).*

Divers Alert Network (DAN): Nonprofit medical, education, and research organization dedicated to the safety and health of scuba divers. www.diversalertnetwork.org

High Altitude Medicine Guide: Current medical information on the prevention, recognition, and treatment of altitude illness, as well as

other health issues affecting travelers to high mountainous regions of the world.
www.high-altitude-medicine.com

International Association for Medical Assistance to Travellers (IAMAT): Provides impartial and accurate travel health advice and coordinates an international network of qualified medical practitioners to assist travelers in need of emergency medical care during a trip.
www.iamat.org

International Society of Travel Medicine: Provides an online and searchable global travel clinic directory.
www.istm.org

MASTA, England: Create your own Travel Health Brief, which a health care professional will use to better understand the risks you may face and help you decide the travel health protection that's right for you.
www.masta-travel-health.com

Medical Advisory Services for Travellers Abroad (MASTA), Australia: Provides professional travel health advice to doctors, pharmacists, pathologists, corporations, government departments, and travel agents; advice available immediately online to subscribers.
www.masta.edu.au

Travel Health ONLINE: Destination information, traveler information, travel medicine providers.
www.tripprep.com

U.S. Department of State: (1) foreign embassy information and publications (www.state.gov/s/cpr/rls); (2) international travel warnings, alerts, and tips (travel.state.gov/travel/travel_1744.html).

World Health Organization (WHO): (1) links for health topics, data and statistics, media center, publications, countries, programs and projects, and about the organization (www.who.int);
(2) *International Travel and Health* guide on health risks for travelers (www.who.int/ith).

Wilderness Medicine: Wilderness and travel medicine conferences, continuing wilderness medicine education.
www.wilderness-medicine.com

INDEX

ABOUT THE AUTHOR

Eric A. Weiss, M.D., F.A.C.E.P., is Associate Professor of Emergency Medicine at Stanford University School of Medicine and Medical Director of the Office of Emergency Management for Stanford Hospital and Lucile Packard Children's Hospital. He is Director of the The Stanford University Fellowship in Wilderness Medicine. Dr. Weiss is a former board member of the Wilderness Medical Society, Chairman of the Wilderness Medical Section of the American College of Emergency Physicians, Medical Director of San Mateo County Emergency Medical Services Agency, and former Medical Editor for *Backpacker Magazine*.

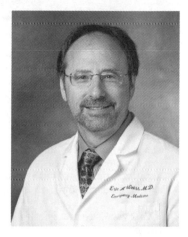

Dr. Weiss is a medical advisor and has been an expedition physician for the National Geographic Society and a medical officer for the Himalayan Rescue Association of Nepal. He has lectured on wilderness and travel medicine to thousands of health care professionals throughout the world and is widely considered the nation's foremost authority on wilderness medicine.

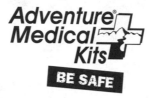

Based in Oakland, California, Adventure Medical Kits (AMK) is one of the largest suppliers of first-aid and survival kits in the world, and is dedicated to delivering the most innovative products which will keep you safe in the outdoors. The AMK team's love of the outdoors is matched only by their drive to create products that allow you to stay healthy on land, water, and air. They rely on the expertise of world authorities in wilderness medicine and survival techniques to develop and refine their products year after year. From comprehensive medical kits for wilderness, marine, and travel adventures, to survival, insect protection, hygiene, foot care, and QuikClot products—AMK keeps you safe and ready for any outdoor adventure.

Visit www.adventuremedicalkits.com for more information and products.

THE MOUNTAINEERS, founded in 1906, is a nonprofit outdoor activity and conservation organization whose mission is "to explore, study, preserve, and enjoy the natural beauty of the outdoors . . . ." Based in Seattle, Washington, it is now one of the largest such organizations in the United States, with seven branches throughout Washington State.

The Mountaineers sponsors both classes and year-round outdoor activities in the Pacific Northwest, which include hiking, mountain climbing, ski-touring, snowshoeing, bicycling, camping, canoeing and kayaking, nature study, sailing, and adventure travel. The Mountaineers' conservation division supports environmental causes through educational activities, sponsoring legislation, and presenting informational programs.

All activities are led by skilled, experienced volunteers, who are dedicated to promoting safe and responsible enjoyment and preservation of the outdoors.

If you would like to participate in these organized outdoor activities or programs, consider a membership in The Mountaineers. For information and an application, write or call The Mountaineers Program Center, 7700 Sand Point Way NE, Seattle, WA 98115-3996; phone 206-521-6001; visit www.mountaineers.org; or email info@mountaineers.org

The Mountaineers Books, an active, nonprofit publishing program of The Mountaineers, produces guidebooks, instructional texts, historical works, natural history guides, and works on environmental conservation. All books produced by The Mountaineers Books fulfill the mission of The Mountaineers. Visit www.mountaineersbooks.org to find details about all our titles and the latest author events, as well as videos, web clips, links, and more!

The Mountaineers Books
1001 SW Klickitat Way, Suite 201
Seattle, WA 98134
800-553-4453
mbooks@mountaineersbooks.org

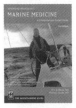
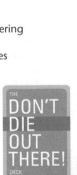
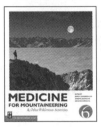
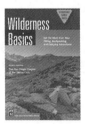